# a guy's
# gotta eat

RUSS KLETTKE
WITH **DEANNA CONTE, M.S., R.D., L.D.**

# a guy's gotta eat

## THE REGULAR GUY'S GUIDE TO EATING SMART

**MARLOWE & COMPANY**
**NEW YORK**

Published by
Marlowe & Company
An Imprint of Avalon Publishing Group Incorporated
245 West 17th Street • 11th Floor
New York, NY 10011-5300

Library of Congress Cataloging-in-Publication Data

Klettke, Russ.
    A guy's gotta eat: the regular guy's guide to eating smart /
    by Russ Klettke and Deanna Conte.
        p. cm.
    Includes index.
    ISBN 1-56924-483-9
    1. Men—Nutrition. 2. Men—Health and hygiene. I. Conte,
    Deanna. II. Title

    RA777.8.K548 2003
    613.2'081—dc21

                                                    2003041296

9  8  7  6  5  4  3  2  1

*Designed by Pauline Neuwirth, Neuwirth & Associates, Inc.*

Printed in the United States of America
Distributed by Publishers Group West

To my mom, Jean Klettke, currently feeding a
fourth generation of Klettke guys.

—Russ Klettke

To the most important men in my life—
my father and my three brothers—
who have provided me with the insight
to truly understand the male of the species.

—Deanna Conte

# contents

*Foreword*                                                    ix

**introduction**                                              xv
*Take Back the Plate*

PART I. **GET SMART**                                          1

**1  a guy's gotta manage his weight**                         3
*Fat, thin, or buff, everyone has a goal—*
*better to achieve it through lifelong habits than*
*a crash program*

**2  a guy's gotta be a caveman**                             23
*To rise to the next level you must first devolve*

**3  a guy's gotta play in the ballpark**                     37
*The math of nutrition*

**4  a guy's gotta eat simple and fast**                      67
*Convenience is greatest at home, and it comes in cans,*
*freezer bags, and a little foresight*

**5  a guy's gotta respect his vices**                        79
*Smart eating doesn't have to be an*
*all-or-nothing proposition*

**6  a guy's gotta eat like a guy**                           87
*Inherent advantages over girls that most guys don't know about*

**7 a guy's gotta eat foods that taste good**     99
*Leverage your favorite flavors to smarter eating*


## PART II. GET EQUIPPED     119

**8 a guy's gotta prep his kitchen**     121
*The essential tools of the cave*

**9 a guy's gotta buy groceries
(but not very often)**     129
*A man's home is his fast-food castle*


## PART III. GET TO WORK     139

**10 a guy's gotta master a few
basics in the kitchen**     141
*Rules of thumb for cooking*

**11 a guy's gotta make a meal
in less than fifteen minutes**     149
*Subsistence cooking for the beginner*

**12 a guy's gotta cook for a date**     183
*Just making the effort can win her heart*

**13 a guy's gotta barbecue**     215
*The care and feeding of friends can be smart, too*


## PART IV. GET OUTTA THE HOUSE     241

**14 a guy's gotta eat out**     243
*Guys eat out more than anyone else—
all the more reason to do it right*

*Bibliography*     273
*Acknowledgments*     279
*Index*     281

# foreword

**I AM THRILLED** to have worked on this book, because I have seen firsthand where healthy eating can succeed and where it can fail. In particular, I believe strongly in finding a way to make "smart" eating both practical and enjoyable.

As a registered dietitian, I've worked in Boston-area hospitals and out-patient counseling centers focused on broad nutrition counseling, health promotion, and weight management. During my graduate work, I was a research assistant on studies that focused on the relationship between food intake and exercise. More recently, I have worked in fitness centers focusing on nutritional counseling, health promotion, wellness, and weight management.

Thanks to my research and practical experience, I have been asked to provide articles and information to a number of media organizations, and have also provided testimony before the Joint Commission on Health Care Oversight hearing on the Boston Marathon.

My clinical experience includes time spent on a cardiothoracic floor, counseling patients (young and old) who had high cholesterol and had gone through heart attacks, angioplasty, and bypass surgery. I also worked on a general medical and surgical floor with diabetic, orthopedic, and arthritic patients, who often required surgical interventions such as kidney transplants, artificial joints, and amputations. Many of these conditions and diseases often directly resulted from, or were exacerbated by, dietary indiscretion and obesity. I spent the last year of my clinical experience working on an oncology floor seeing individuals with all types of cancers—a majority of whom, I'm sad to say, did not survive. We now know that many cancers are directly linked to dietary factors and body weight. The diets I recommended were intended to keep the patients strong throughout their treatment. This included helping patients contend with the unpleasant and debilitating effects of chemotherapy and radiation.

While treating patients who were already inflicted with a disease or disorder, it became clear to me that I would rather focus on prevention, before diseases develop and significant medical management becomes necessary. In 1998, I began to switch gears and to focus on education, weight loss, counseling, fitness, and wellness.

I now help clients establish a sense of balance in their lives. Their goals include losing weight, living longer, being more productive, having more energy, and improving their health. But most seem not to know where to start. Many individuals have high levels of stress, and spend a great deal of time working, eating on the go, dining outside of the home, and traveling— all factors that tend to cause poor dietary intake.

By the time these clients come in to see me, almost all of them describe having tried several different programs in the past. They have read books on health, wellness, and weight loss. But they all describe virtually the same experience: a general feeling of failure and of confusion, an overall negative experience. Not exactly a recipe for success.

After working with nutrition clients as a nutritionist and registered dietitian for the past eight years, my philosophy is to incorporate small but consistent lifestyle changes that a person can live with, without feeling deprived, backed into a corner, or that they must eat things that just don't taste good. This starts with education and empowerment—and never losing sight of the fact that eating should be enjoyable, even fun.

I'm also seeing more male clients than in the past. It has become clear that men have different needs than women—guys simply have a different way of approaching things. One thing I've found is that guys are able to make improvements one step at a time.

*A Guy's Gotta Eat* is designed specifically to meet men's needs. It is a smart, simple, no-nonsense, non-dieting approach that we know healthy and fit people generally follow intuitively. It's nutritionally sound, well balanced, and, most importantly, there's no food you cannot eat (in moderation). Even pizza, hamburgers, and ice cream! It's also fun and easy—

with coaching on everything from how to stock your kitchen with the necessary utensils and what to buy at the grocery store, to grilling and preparing meals in less than fifteen minutes. It's this practical approach, establishing healthy habits you can live with, that will make the difference between success and failure.

A *Guy's Gotta Eat* is a great tool—one that every guy should have in his toolbox!

*Deanna Conte, M.S., R.D., L.D.*

# a guy's gotta eat

# introduction

## Take back the plate

**It's a weird** time to be a guy with an appetite. The world of healthy eating just doesn't seem to be programmed for us. Wherever we go, our convenience-food culture—fast food, convenience stores, gas-and-go dining, pizza deliveries—allows us to grab a quick fix, morning, noon, and night. And, being guys, we're busy. We have jobs, we work out and play sports (maybe), we commute hither and yon, we like to get together with our friends. We watch TV. We don't have much time to shop or cook.

Yet today, more so than a generation ago, there is a lot of pressure on us to be healthy, look good, perform enthusiastically, and be smart. We know that eating right affects all of these needs. But most guys can't see how they're supposed to maintain good nutrition in a fast and crazy world. It's a strange paradox that all adults in industrialized countries, guys included, are more overweight and less healthy at younger ages than ever before.

*A Guy's Gotta Eat* takes a different look at this whole equation. If you're a guy, and particularly if you're single, you have a couple of key advantages in the quest to maintain good nutrition. First, you have more control over your circumstances than people who cohabitate with partners and/or children. Second, I'll make a broad generalization and suggest that guys, by and large, are creatures of habit. We like most of what we do and we stick with it. We tend to work well with a certain degree of structure.

The quality of your nutritional structure might be the defining difference between you and me. I—and about fifty other guys interviewed for this book—have a good structure. But you probably don't. I've set up my life so that when I'm hungry, I eat what is most convenient and appealing. It just happens to be smart food, too. My structure differs from how the majority of people live today. When I arrive home after a long day, I can whip together a great-tasting, nutritious meal in less than fifteen minutes. We know from food-product consumption data that many other people, especially guys, get their dinner at a drive-through, from a frozen entrée, or delivered.

It's not as if you don't see the error of your ways, at least in some vague sense. You *have* had a few healthy meals—say, savory chicken with lemon-garlic broccoli and wild rice. You probably know that it beats frozen chicken potpies and pizza for nutritional value as well as taste. Now imagine that you made that meal yourself in under fifteen minutes, about half the time required to thaw and bake the potpie, and a third the time needed for a pizza delivery. I'm not talking about a frozen, packaged entrée, either. You can do it if you have a structure—know-how and the correct utensils and foods—right there in your kitchen, ready when you are hungry. For the times you eat out—about half of American meals are prepared out of the home—you might like to know the simple differences between smart and dumb menu choices. Whether at home or away, the most surprising result of the healthy-eating structure in this book is that it is faster, easier, more economical, and tastier than most convenience food.

Note also that this book, like many others on the topic of eating and health, discusses body fat and obesity. These are not the only measures or indicators of health. There are thin people who eat poorly and may suffer negative health consequences as a result. There are very muscular people who have made building muscle a singular goal—to the exclusion of long-term well-being (this includes guys who consider protein bars to be a complete meal).

The key principles of this book steer you toward adopting simple, basic eating habits that can be beneficial into old age. These principles apply to all types of people—men, women, the physically active, and people who have yet to take up exercise. But *A Guy's Gotta Eat* builds a structure that most likely will work for single guys, helping you overcome obstacles and capitalize on opportunities that your married and female friends don't have.

## THIS CAN BE EASY

LET'S START WITH THE good news. Eating smart doesn't have to be hard. Preparing good food at home—or finding nutritious stuff outside of the home—doesn't need to take up a lot of time. Make-at-home meals in this book take only a third of the time that it takes for a standard pizza delivery (fifteen minutes versus forty-five minutes). As for grocery shopping, it's possible to limit it to once a month because some of the smartest foods out there are frozen or canned, or will keep fresh for several weeks. (Reread that last sentence. Frozen and canned foods are good for you; in fact, they usually have more nutrients than fresh foods. More on that later.)

More good news: Good eating works best when it's pleasurable. When healthier food tastes good, you're more likely to eat it instead of things like fried cheese sticks and sugar-coated pastries. Taste—mouthwatering, succulent, satisfying flavor—is a high priority of this book.

Your first big steps to improvement can happen in a single day—or you can chip away at it gradually, if that's how you like to work.

I decided to write this book because I see too many people agonizing over simple matters of food and nutrition. With a little bit of study, the choices involved become simple, the process easy. Going out on a limb, I dare even say it can be fun.

If you find this surprising, perhaps it's because most books and other media coverage on the topic are not written with single guys in mind.

Consequently, you may not pay attention to discussion of nutrition and cooking. All that noise in the media about nutrition bores you, confuses you, or ignores your needs and interests. Articles called "Thinner Thighs by the Fourth of July" do not inspire you to go out and buy a vegetable steamer. "Quick Tips for Preventing Alzheimer's with Berries" might not hit home, either. You have to search high and low for an article like "Vegetables That Make You a Better Man," and then it might disappoint you that tomatoes only indirectly benefit virility and mainly prevent prostate cancer (this is ultimately of consequence to your manhood, but is not the natural Viagra you wanted). And when you run across a recipe that has twenty ingredients and requires soaking something overnight, you'll probably check out right there.

You can't be blamed for not paying attention—you're a busy guy with a lot going on in your life. So why make the effort? For starters, take a look at the statistics. American adults, including single men as much as women, seniors, and children, are getting fat like there's no tomorrow. More than 60 percent of adults (and 14 percent of adolescents) are overweight or obese. And it's getting worse fast. According to the *Journal of the American Medical Association,* between 1991 and 1998 the number of obese men in the 18–29 age bracket increased by *almost 70 percent.*

Gentlemen, clearly we have a problem. *Three hundred thousand* people die each year from illnesses caused by excess weight, according to U.S. Surgeon General David Satcher. Health-care costs are going to climb over the next several decades because 68 percent of modern illnesses are caused or made worse by bad diets. A majority of overweight Americans don't exercise, but even among those who do, they're still eating mountains of (unhealthy) foods that probably shouldn't have been invented in the first place.

It's time for guys to discover how smart eating is very simple and mindlessly convenient. Maybe your incentive to eat smarter is not about weight control. It might be to increase muscle mass, or just improve vitality, or you have your eyes on long-term health issues. With a just a little variation, the path to each of these results is basically the same.

## SMART FOOD IS EVERYWHERE (and so is the dumb stuff)

FOR ANY GUY WHO thinks, *I should eat better,* it is the best of times and it is the worst of times. It's a tale of two tables. Things are not entirely your fault—it's easy to be drawn to bad food choices. One of the biggest forces that determine which foods are most available to you—the food industry—has complicated the simple matter of food and eating. Food and beverage manufacturers have introduced 116,000 new products to U.S. consumers since 1990. Some are good for us, some clearly are not, and many either make misleading health claims—"fat free" has become a cover for foods loaded with refined sugar—or are detrimental when eaten in excess.

From a best-of-times perspective, there has never been more information available on how to eat right. Doctors and researchers are learning and reporting more every day about foods and diets that contribute to better health; while these programs are often pitted against each other— for example, the Atkins diet versus the Zone diet versus the government's food pyramid—in many ways they are similar and provide us with information from which to work. Along with that, there have never been more foods to help a guy improve his health, maintain his preferred weight, and allow him the energy to work, play, and generally enjoy his life. Good examples are prepeeled and washed carrots and leaf lettuce, sold in plastic bags and ready to eat, and frozen chicken breasts in ziplock bags that allow you to cook them one at a time. Everything you need is out there.

But this is where the problem starts. All that information and all these choices inspire some wacky ideas and moronic food inventions (such as chicken "nuggets" covered in batter and deep-fried so that what started out healthy ends up as a nutrition failure). Countering the plain, clear sense that foods closest to the farm are the best for us—vegetables, fruit, dairy, lean meat, whole grains—are contradictory ideas from a cast of characters selling books and appearing in the media. They either say we can eat all the bacon and fried chicken we want (but should never, ever eat another piece of bread), or, on the opposite end of the spectrum, there are extremists who would rather we graze our way gently through prairies untouched by modern agriculture. Meanwhile, there's another segment of experts (and their books) that would have us fasting, drinking vinegar, and completely avoiding whole categories of food (such as eggs, milk, meat, or wheat), even when we have no medical condition that requires it. And then there's the food supplementation industry, making money off questionable science and vitamins and herbs never subjected to valid scientific research. So if you haven't been paying attention, don't worry. A lot of it is hooey—or at the very least, small chunks of information presented out of context that make this whole business unnecessarily complicated.

## AN AGGRESSIVE CONVENIENCE CULTURE

FOR A LITTLE PERSPECTIVE, just take a long, hard look at the way large segments of the food industry pursue your wallet and stomach. Foods with little to no nutritional value are being aggressively marketed and distributed so that you can dine on them during long work commutes or within the comforts of your home or workplace. The convenience-food industry knows who you are and where to find you. In fact, if there is a single perpetrator of unhealthy eating it's our convenience culture. We've somehow been convinced that a quick meal or snack is an entitlement with no consequences. The food industry has ingeniously stepped forward with products made to be eaten while in transit, even to the point of being purchased without leaving our cars (roughly half of fast-food sales at major chains are at the drive-through). Most of these products are made from agricultural goods whose native nutrients are processed out of them months before they reach your digestive system. Most entice us with fatty, salty, or sugary flavors. A vast majority (but not all) of convenience foods have a negative impact on our health, vitality, and looks.

And single guys are sitting ducks. Look at how they market to us: An April 2001 press release from Jack in the Box restaurants crows, "We discovered that our target audience, men ages 18–43, want more meat and cheese. So we designed the Triple Ultimate Cheeseburger for cheeseburger purists who don't want a salad on their burger." Nice—they're going after us with a single meal that provides 990 calories, 66 grams of fat, and a measly 2 grams of fiber—roughly 103 percent of the recommended daily intake of fat. I guess you're supposed to gnaw on celery for the next twenty-four hours. Across the street, Burger King uses comedian/personality Adam Carolla of *The Man Show* as its commercial pitchman. Pepsi is spending $200 million for a five-year contract as the official soft drink of the National Football League, while Coke shelled out $500 million for its eleven-year sponsorship of the National Collegiate Athletic Association. They're clearly making money by selling you brownish bubbly sugar water. Certainly there are women who pump their own gas, but in your gut you know that most of the food sold in gas-station convenience stores—chips and candies crowd aisles to last the miles—are consumed by men.

# WHO WANTS YOU?

IT'S NOT TOO hard to see the correlation between which companies spend the most to advertise and what ends up in your mouth—after all, without your purchases they couldn't afford the billions spent on commercials. By brand value—cumulative consumer recognition, a function of marketing expenditure—here's the top ten worldwide ranking of food, beverage, and tobacco companies in 2001:

> **1.** Coca-Cola (food/beverages)
> **2.** McDonald's (food retail)
> **3.** Marlboro (tobacco)
> **4.** Nescafé (beverages)
> **5.** Heinz (food)
> **6.** Budweiser (alcohol)
> **7.** Kellogg's (food/beverages)
> **8.** Pepsi-Cola (beverages)
> **9.** Wrigley's (food)
> **10.** Bacardi (alcohol)

> Source: Interbrand, a market-tracking firm, as reported in Russell Ash's *The Top 10 of Everything,* 2002, DK Publishing, Inc., 2001.

No wonder Americans are getting butts and guts like watermelons. Diseases that were far less common a century ago—diabetes, certain cancers, and even heart diseases—are now epidemic. Information and choices seem not to have helped much. For the overweight, obese, and unhealthy, life really must present some paradoxes. They see television commercials starring swimsuited hardbodies swilling beer and playing volleyball, jumping into sports cars, or just smelling swell; thirty seconds later they're told the whole time-pressed family should eat sugar-infused snack cakes for breakfast.

## GUYS GOTTA BE GUYS

GO ON, ADMIT IT. If given the choice between a Victoria's Secret model and that really fun girl in your freshman English composition class with a shapeless body, you'd much rather spend an evening discussing the challenges of runway work than the hazards of run-on sentences. If you're gay, you want to know if the model has an available brother. That's because you're a guy. And guys are guys. It's built into our genes to seek out the most healthy, nubile thing out there in order to propagate the species. As the spreader of seeds, it's a guy's job to find the fields offering the best yields. You are simply true to your nature.

The funny thing is, Mr. Farmer, the models *and* lit majors have a say in the matter too. It ain't the caveman days any more—you can't just grab *objet d'affection* by the ponytail and drag her back to some warm spot. They've come a long way, baby. They want you to be as buff as the guys in the shaving ads. You might hate that, or conversely you may be deluded into thinking that you are just as hot as the televised towel-clad guy caressing his smooth face.

But here's where it still *is* the caveman days. Our bodies evolved over time to exist on foods that were available through nature, including times such as winter, drought, monsoons, and infestations, when food was short. Our forebears ate right from the tree, stalks in the field, tubers from the ground, fish from the river, and beasts they could knock out with a rock (humans were initially scavengers, eating the leftovers from other animals). No company or cook got in their way, and our digestive system processed nutrients best in that fashion.

Fast-forward to the twenty-first century. Our stomach, pancreas, liver, and other organs involved in nutrient absorption are facing Ho Hos and colas. Maybe for breakfast. It might taste good but, for the love of God, pay attention to what it's doing to your body.

Beyond matters of weight control, if you're eating processed, high-fat and -calorie foods, chances are there's no room left in your stomach for foods with health-promoting properties. A meal based in French fries nudges a side of vegetables off the plate; cheesecake does the same thing to a bowl of raspberries. Vegetables and fruit, fresh and frozen, are packed with micronutrients that help your body and brain work best and fight disease. Your body has evolved to make use of plant foods and lean protein; without these things, you are bucking nature. This is a very key point. A lot of guys need to lose weight, but others simply want to eat healthier. These are the two sides of the same coin—eat smarter (healthier) so there's less room for the dumber things (which cause unwanted weight gain). Make it a habit and excess weight, if you have any, is far more likely to disappear.

The fact is that if you want to live a better life, you gotta take back the plate. Make what goes into your mouth your own smart choice. Part of that is knowing how to avert the convenience culture. It's no harder—and probably less expensive—than what you're doing currently.

## MANAGING YOUR HEALTH THROUGH SMART EATING

*A GUY'S GOTTA EAT* IS not written for most people. This book does not address the needs and lifestyles of women, seniors, children, and responsible father/husband types who eat in family settings. It's about how single guys can and should eat—about half the time at home, the other half out of the home—because we have greater independence and control over our gastronomic domain. If you like foods such as peanut butter on bananas or chicken made with steak sauce, this is the place for you. If you like to eat directly from the jar, no plate involved, this book respects your right to do that. In fact, I even encourage it. Even if you absolutely must eat a whole pizza all by yourself once in a while (I do), you've come to the right place. Most importantly, this book is about fighting back against the dumb, twisted products that the convenience-food industry throws at you without any regard to your needs: to be fit, to feel great, and to perform better. And it is meant to establish habits that will improve your odds at fighting off heart disease, certain cancers, and diabetes as you age. And note that the onset of such diseases can be as early as the mid–thirties, in part from bad dietary habits established at younger ages. Epidemiologists note an up-tick in many diet-related diseases among people under age forty, most likely due to the obesity epidemic affecting adolescents and young adults.

# LINK BETWEEN OBESITY AND CANCER IN MEN

**A** SIXTEEN-YEAR STUDY of 900,000 Americans found that men have a 52 percent greater chance of dying from cancer if they are overweight. By that math, one in six cancer deaths could be prevented by weight management—about 90,000 people per year. The following are linked to excess weight:

Colon cancer

Prostate cancer

Esophageal cancer

Kidney cancer

Stomach cancer

Liver cancer

Pancreatic cancer

Non-Hodgkin's lymphoma

Multiple myeloma

Rectal cancer

Gall bladder cancer

Source: American Cancer Society (Eugenia Calle, director of analytic epidemiology and lead author of the study, 2003).

## HOW MY APPROACH IS DIFFERENT

IN THE INTEREST OF full disclosure, let me share with you my background in food and health. First, I am not a nutritionist or dietitian. That's why Deanna Conte, registered dietitian, has reviewed and advised on every last word of this book. Deanna is a rare find—she's one of the few dietitians who is engaged daily in the relationship between exercise and nutrition (she counsels health club members and was a competitive swimmer in high school and college). Her academic and clinical training qualifies her to validate my approach. When she meets with members at The Sports Club/LA in Boston, her place of employment, she is witness to the common nutrition misunderstandings of both men and women. "They really need this," she told me when I first approached her about helping out with the book. "A lot of people are so unaware." (Another interesting irony in the face of America's obesity epidemic is that health club memberships are at an all-time high. People want to improve their bodies, but half the equation, eating, is given far less attention in most gyms.)

Second, I've never formally studied cooking, except for interviews with professional cooks as part of my research for this book, and perusal of related books, magazines, and television programs. I once microwaved a steak (it doesn't work; it turned out gray and too chewy). When I entertain, I con my friends into helping me in the kitchen (some of their best ideas are in this book). I frugally eat at home more often than many of my peers, and I typically experiment with healthier foods to find ways I can enjoy them. This book delivers an accumulation of my best discoveries over twenty years of living single, keeping myself fed and fit.

And my life is atypical. You'll find me at the gym between four and six times a week, a discipline rooted in years on my high school swim team. I truly enjoy most forms of exercise. And when I'm not at the gym, I'm training on a bike, running, or swimming—in fact, I've competed in more than thirty triathlons since 1987, and intend to continue as long as possible. I live in Chicago, where I can reach a majority of the places I need to go—work, the gym, stores, social events—on one of my two bikes. Also, I've been interested in nutrition and health since I was a kid, reading articles like "I Am Joe's Liver" in *Reader's Digest* back in the 1960s, which was pretty weird at the time but something I now appreciate. In the years since, I've read hundreds of reports on the relationship between diet, exercise, and general health. I also worked in food service in college, and have held positions in public relations for several food companies, including McDonald's Corporation's public relations firm and The NutraSweet Company. I have never been overweight, although I see my weight fluctuate yearly by about ten pounds, usually due to the seasonal nature of triathlon training. I can also tell you how hard it is for me to stop at a single portion of potato chips (vinegar-salt flavor) or ice cream (peanut butter) when I have such things around the house.

So why write a book? It started with a friendly business lunch a few years ago with a guy named Brian. God bless him; Brian is well aware of many things in life, but nutrition just isn't one of them. He works out and clearly has fitness goals. But at that lunch he talked about his inability to drop about ten pounds as he stabbed one fried potato after the other from his plate. I outlined a nutrition primer on a napkin while he peppered me with questions on the practicality of cooking regularly and grocery shopping, in addition to telling me how he wouldn't eat tofu salad in restaurants. It was then that I realized my accumulated knowledge and somewhat pragmatic approach to all this was something that guys like Brian could use. He needed more than just information—he had to be shown a realistic way to incorporate smart eating into his life.

To supplement our own experience, Deanna and I conducted a series of straw polls among friends and colleagues as a test of our own perceptions of what guys deal with when it comes to nutrition and weight management. *A Guy's Gotta Eat* is a distillation of all our experiences and those of about one hundred other people, as well as the smart findings of weight management and nutrition experts all over the world. The result is *informed common sense* on how single men can practically manage their overall health, including their weight.

*A Guy's Gotta Eat* is laid out in four parts. Part I takes you through points on weight management and explains how nutrition is a function of our evolution, how single guys are uniquely equipped to eat smart, and why you need to prioritize good-tasting food. Part II is about how to buy the equipment and groceries that can make your home a healthy eating environment, while Part III shows you how to put those purchases to work. The final section of the book shows you smart ways to spend the approximate half of all food dollars most single men spend eating outside the home.

# PART I

# GET SMART

**HAVE YOU** ever wondered why there are so many different theories on weight loss and weight management? It's because no one knows for sure. In part, that results from the difficulty of measuring the interplay between eating behaviors, activity levels, genetic variations between individuals, and the differences between men and women. What works for some might not work for others, and few studies honestly track behaviors beyond a year or two. All of this suggests that the individual is responsible for finding his own best approach.

All this attention to weight loss has at least helped uncover some reasonably sound advice. For example, all the theories agree that we need to reduce our consumption of processed foods—things sold in boxes, bags, and cans, in geometric shapes and colors not known in nature, such as Lucky Charms, goldfish crackers, and colas. It's better to eat meat, poultry, fish, grains, and produce, foods that look a lot like they did back on the farm, on the ranch, or in the sea.

A Guy's Gotta Eat illustrates the conveniences of smart food in the twenty-first century. You will have to learn a few things and develop a few basic skills, but if you have that nagging sense that you should be eating better, this is the place to learn how.

This section lays out the scientific component of how food functions, both biologically and socially. This includes understanding food relative to human evolution, how we function with excess, how to source and store food within time limitations, getting perspective on indulgences, and how being a guy affects how we eat and even how we taste our food, all within the practical realities of guyhood. Strangely, food and eating have gotten way too complicated. If you want to eat smart, it will help to understand some simple facts about how our bodies deal with food.

First, we'll take a guy-centric look at the thing on almost everyone's mind: weight.

**1**

# a guy's gotta manage his weight

## Fat, thin, or buff, everyone has a goal—better to achieve it through lifelong habits than a crash program

**If you eat** smart, you shouldn't have to diet. I'll repeat that: Eating smart = no dieting. That's what perpetually fit and healthy people do. They naturally eat every meal, every day with an eye on health. It's ingrained in their habits and their life so much that meals and snacks are subconscious decisions, not a matter of self-denial or deprivation. In fact, truly healthy people who understand food probably enjoy their meals more than those who don't.

*A Guy's Gotta Eat* should help you achieve perpetual fitness and health, as much as mortal condition allows. You'll understand food so you can select items in grocery stores, on restaurant menus, and from your own refrigerator that are going to serve your better health interests. Further, you'll know how to make food taste so good that you'll look forward to your own cooking.

How does that work? First, educate yourself. The fact that you're reading this book suggests that you understand that much. Second, take stock of the advantages you have, as a guy in the twenty-first century, in controlling what you eat—there's never been more access to great food and technology that can make you the master of your dinner plate. Third, acknowledge that you need to put a little time and money into it. But note that this is no more time and money than you already spend on food, even if you're routinely a fast-food, drive-through diner. You will save both time and money if you get smart about food.

## WEIGHT MANAGEMENT VERSUS WEIGHT LOSS

TAKE A LOOK THROUGH the magazine racks and Web sites that carry health information. You might get the idea that everyone needs to lose weight. The truth of the matter is that more than 60 percent of American adults do—guys more so than women. About 20 percent of us are seriously overweight, technically obese, and in danger of life-threatening health problems (diabetes, heart disease, and cancer, for starters).

But even buff-looking people might be unhealthy. Super-thin people quite often get that way by consciously starving themselves, exercising maniacally, smoking cigarettes, or worse. The worlds of professional sports, Olympic athletics, and competitive bodybuilding are well known to be populated with users and abusers of steroids and other illegal performance-enhancing drugs. Such individuals court long-term health problems, including premature death. Several amateur and professional athletes have died in sports training in recent years due to the use of ephedra and other stimulants in attempts to either lose weight or achieve other physical ideals. Meanwhile, high school athletes look to use the same shortcuts to physical achievement. That's insane.

But almost as crazy as that is what modern conveniences and food-product marketing have done to our food. A confluence of technology, economics and free enterprise, social pressures, and simple inattention are largely responsible for the health mismanagement that is occurring through broad swaths of our society.

Your objective should be maximum health for the long term. That would include managing your weight and increasing your odds of avoiding disease in the future. Unlike supermodels and other legend wannabes, most reasonable people want to achieve a set point of physical equilibrium, usually a specific body weight and degree of muscularity. The better term for this is *weight management*. This might mean gaining pounds for some, losing for many others, or just shifting weight around from one area (for example, the stomach) to another (the shoulders). Exercise, including physical activity that comes with daily living and some occupations, will always play a central role in weight management. But what we eat plays an equally important function.

To get a sense of what average guys think of food and their health, I quizzed about fifty people I know, most in relatively good health, a majority of whom belong to a gym and maintain their weight. Almost all of them had reached a point in their lives where they decided to adjust their eating and workout patterns to improve their physique and health. Here is a sampling of what they said:

> I saw that I've put on about fifteen pounds since I got out of college (eight years ago). After turning thirty-one, it became more clear that I wasn't getting away with eating crap like before (e.g., ice cream almost every night).
> — *Tom, Chicago, Illinois*

> I changed my eating habits when I started working out on a consistent basis.
> — *Keith, Chicago, Illinois*

> I had a heart attack at age thirty-nine. I realized I needed to be protective around my eating. I was fit and trim before my heart attack, but a lot of travel on the road led to unhealthy eating habits. It all caught up with me, and I got sick.
> — *John, Chicago, Illinois*

I used to weigh three hundred pounds with a forty-seven-inch waist. I got tired of feeling bad physically and emotionally.

—*Jay, San Diego, California*

Once you turn forty that "I can eat anything and not gain a pound" reality is *gone.* It takes a couple of years for that to sink in and then you either head down that path to a thirty-eight-inch waist or change your habits.

—*Chris, San Francisco, California*

Aspen, February 5th, 2001. I couldn't fit into my father's ski pants.

—*Jeff, Washington, D.C.*

Marriage. High cholesterol diagnosis (228 in 1994, now 180).

—*Stu, Austin, Texas*

I needed to eat more calories and specifically more protein to gain muscle while working out.

—*Jason, Fort Lauderdale, Florida*

Throughout *A Guy's Gotta Eat,* the principles and practices outlined should be applicable to all three weight-management strategies—to lose, to gain, or to maintain. How can the same regimen work so magically for different people with different goals? *A Guy's Gotta Eat* isn't exactly a regimen. It's more of a *leaning,* consisting of ways of thinking, tips, good advice, practical how-to instruction, reference information to answer frequent questions, and things you can do that, if you're not doing them already, will bring about positive change.

Sorry if that disappoints you. If you want a step-by-step schedule with absolute mandates, there are other books, Web sites, and classes that provide that. If you want to pack on twenty or more pounds of muscle, you need a personal trainer and books on bodybuilding. If you are looking to lose a significant amount of weight, this probably would still work, because it's about getting rid of the bad habits that likely contributed to your present condition. But always seek supervision from a qualified professional such as a doctor or dietitian who can identify the complete set of factors affecting your weight.

Keep in mind that weight "loss" and "gain" goals cannot effectively be accomplished through food alone. Physical activity—whether it be a structured exercise program or just simply opting out of labor-saving devices like golf carts (walk), elevators (take the stairs), short car rides (bike), and hired housekeepers or gardeners (do it yourself)—will always play a role.

If you're seeking to maintain your weight and are primarily interested in staving off diseases through healthier eating, you may not need to increase the amount of exercise you do—assuming you are physically active to begin with. Exercise should always be a part of a guy's life, even into old age.

In all three strategies—losing, gaining, and maintaining—train your eye toward the long term. Do you think health and fitness are important only at your current age? Ask someone five, ten, or twenty years older than you. How you feel and look becomes more important, and often more challenging, for people as time goes on (except for those who give up). Body weight isn't the only factor affecting overall health. Your ability to stave off disease, which can be *significantly* affected by micronutrients in foods, becomes more critical as you age.

Let's talk about the word *diet*. Most guys don't use it. We say we're "trying to get in shape." When we use the word here it's about the *structure* of food intake, not the common definition of deprivation and short-term goals. Which brings back the subject of diets. The Atkins diet. The Zone diet. The South Beach diet. Pritikin, Scarsdale, grapefruit, Jenny Craig, and Weight Watchers. Don't they work?

Sure, there are millions of people who've lost weight on these diets. Many have kept off the pounds, and many have not. Guys, let's just learn from their hard work. Each of these diets has revealed important components of human physiology and psychology. Some of that learning is incorporated in this book. And we should thank them all for enlightening us through their trial and error.

Most of these diets are pretty much driven by the idea of weight loss. In particular, the Zone diet (and, to a lesser extent, Atkins) informs this book. It highlights the evolutionary development of humans and how modern food systems largely depart from the way nature intends for us to eat. Adjusting these principles to the pragmatic realities of guy life, we suggest the following strategies for weight management:

## GUYS' TOP TEN PRACTICAL WEIGHT-MANAGEMENT STRATEGIES

### STRATEGY #1: EAT AT HOME MORE OFTEN

According to a report published in the *Journal of the American Dietetic Association* (August 2001), a meal in a restaurant typically contains 55 percent more calories than what one eats at home. Why? They have to entice you with easy-to-achieve-on-a-mass-scale tastes, generally involving grease (oil or lard), salt, and sugar. To illustrate, just note also how many places serve some version of fried potatoes.

Do the math: Say you get dinner three nights a week from a fast-service restaurant and twice a week at a sit-down place. If you learn how to cook just two healthy meals, *just two,* you can cut out the calories of one entire meal each week. Let's say it's two fast-food dinners that you're losing—conservatively, a net reduction of 800 calories per week (probably more)—that could add up to a loss of a 7.6 pounds in a year. You'll eat the same number of meals as before, so there's no deprivation involved.

The bulk of this book provides ideas and guidelines that will enable even the non-cook to learn basic skills of healthy meal preparation. Chapter 3 examines the false economies of "convenience foods"—quite often, it takes more time to get a burger or pizza than to make your own balanced meals at home. With the right equipment and a little skill development, you can learn how to spontaneously toss together a dinner in under fifteen minutes.

Realistically speaking, particularly if you travel a lot for work, you will still need to eat out of the house a third to half of the time. Part IV is included to guide you through fast-food or restaurant meals to your best advantage.

### STRATEGY #2: REDUCE CONSUMPTION OF SIMPLE CARBOHYDRATES

The Atkins diet, the Zone diet, DASH (Dietary Approaches to Stop Hypertension, a research-based approach sponsored by the National Heart, Blood, and Lung Institute), and the South Beach diet all share a significant viewpoint: For various reasons, simple (a.k.a. processed)* carbohydrates

---

*Technically speaking, the sugars in fruit are simple (monosaccharides and disaccharides). But eaten with non-digestible fiber that naturally occurs with whole fruit, the sugar is more slowly digested and therefore is kinder to your blood sugar levels. This is the difference between eating an apple and drinking apple juice.

need to be removed from your meals and snacks as much as possible. This is now considered conventional wisdom in the world of dietary science.

Atkins adherents also say that almost all carbs should be minimized; this book (and others) takes an opposite position. Complete carb avoidance is largely impractical and nearly impossible to maintain outside of laboratory environments. I also concur with those who believe it dangerously discounts the fact that there are two very different kinds of carbohydrates, complex and simple. Just as important, it ignores the significant health benefits of plant food. Understand the differences and you can go a long way toward both weight management and disease prevention.

### Complex Carbohydrates (i.e., Plant Food)

These are the things that *would* become simple (processed) carbs if sent through the mill, mixer, masher, or oven: fruits, vegetables, and whole grains, wild or brown rice, all close to the form they grew in. In whole form, they are more slowly digested and have more nutrients left in them, including vitamins and minerals as well as antioxidants such as beta carotene and vitamin C. Many vegetables contain lycopene, which is an outstanding phytochemical with antioxidant properties. Slower digestion has many benefits, including a noticeable reduction of the fatigue that one feels after a high-carb meal.

Based on extensive research, the National Cancer Institute so believes in the value of fruits and vegetables that they recommend that men eat *nine* servings per day (women are urged to eat seven)—even more than the five-a-day recommendations of the past several years. For example, recent discoveries on the beneficial effects of lycopene (in tomatoes) in preventing prostate cancer should be incentive enough; the ongoing spate of discoveries on plant-based micronutrients suggests we will discover additional benefits from fruits and vegetables in the future.

Fruits and vegetables are at the core of smart eating for several reasons, explored at length throughout this book. Not only do they deliver their own goods, but by filling you up they leave little room for more calorie- and fat-dense foods in your stomach—a key weight-management tactic.

In the modern world, we're unlikely to visit a farm stand every day. So practically speaking we get complex carbs in the next-best form: frozen, canned, or dried fruits and vegetables, which retain some or all of the benefits of their fresh counterparts.

Complex carbs carry calories—some (such as an average banana at 130 calories) much more than others (such as a small peach, 37 calories)—so even they have limits. Some vegetables are extremely low in calories: Per serving, broccoli is about 25 calories, onions between 20 and 30 calories per serving. Extra calories in any form convert to fat if you don't expend them through activity or metabolism, but that's least likely to happen with fruits and vegetables. It's hard to get fat on peaches. Relative to the nutrient benefit, fruits and vegetables could hardly be a better deal.

A lot of guys act like bratty little kids when it comes to vegetables ("I don't *like* cauliflower"). So how do you change that? Find a vegetable you can love. Or at least are willing to date. Find eight ways to flavor it. Once you've experimented with all eight, get produce-promiscuous with a second vegetable. Repeat.

Not sure what you can love? Ask a red cabbage to go home with you. It's cheap, versatile, has an interesting taste and a great texture (almost like pasta), is easy to keep on hand, is filling, and is really low in calories and high in nutrients. Steam, boil, or stir-fry it, flavor it with a little butter and lemon juice. Or make it without butter. Make it sassy with hot sauce, curry, crushed nuts, chopped onion, cholesterol-free bacon bits, and Parmesan cheese.

You could try the same thing with broccoli (frozen, chopped). As a cruciferous vegetable (along with cauliflower, cabbage, watercress, brussels sprouts, and bok choy), broccoli is one of the best vegetables you can eat. A 2002 study in the *Journal of the National Cancer Institute* shows that three or more servings of cruciferous vegetables a week slashes the risk of prostate cancer almost in half. The study involved more than six hundred men with prostate cancer and confirms data from a similar Canadian study showing that cruciferous vegetables, tomatoes, green vegetables, beans, lentils, and nuts all substantially reduce the risk of that common male cancer.

Whole-grain products—whole-grain breads, crackers, pastas, and wild or brown rice, for example—deliver nutrients and fiber. Individuals looking for quick weight loss might follow the No White Carbs (NWC) variations offered in chapter 11; however, that strategy would be better applied to the reduction of simple carbohydrates.

### Simple (Processed) Carbohydrates

Simple carbohydrates begin their lives as plant foods, but are commercially processed into so much less. The result is anything with sugar (most desserts and sweet beverages), as well as baked goods that are not whole grain, made instead with refined flour (white breads, muffins, donuts, pie crusts, pizza crusts, pancakes). White table sugar and high-fructose corn syrup (used in most sweet beverages) are also processed from their origins as sugar cane, corn, or beets. Peeled potatoes (and their progeny, French fries and mashed potatoes), peeled apples, and white rice each have their fibrous, vitamin-rich outer layer removed. They're often referred to as "white carbs" because they've been refined by the removal of other plant components of color. A prime example is white bread.

One way to distinguish simple from complex carbohydrates is to consider how much technology has been used between field and fork: Does the product look like it was just picked, or did it run through a mill, mixer, masher, or oven before it got to you? Note that *whole-grain* bread and pasta are still milled, mixed, mashed, baked, and wrapped in a plastic bag, but at least all components of the grain (bran, endosperm, and germ) remain.

What's taken out in processing of simple carbohydrates—skin, husks, hulls, seeds—would slow the absorption of their natural sugars (fructose); this allows each to be more readily digested, but causes a quick response by your insulin-producing pancreas. This effect is given a score in something called the "glycemic index," which provides relative numbers on how quickly certain foods are absorbed into the bloodstream (slower is better). The end result is that you're hungry again sooner and will be less likely to be physically active—the "bonk" that happens in late afternoon that might dissuade you from an evening run or trip to the gym. In other words, simple carbohydrates have nearly the opposite effect of complex carbs. Learn the distinctions and you'll make significant progress toward weight management.

## STRATEGY #3: INCREASE CONSUMPTION OF LEAN PROTEIN

Supplementing the benefits of complex carbohydrates is protein, which is an essential part of building and maintaining muscle (the benefit of which is detailed in Strategy #4, below). For the record, protein derives primarily from red meat, fish, pork, chicken and turkey, dairy products, eggs, and plant foods such as legumes (beans and soy).

Conventional wisdom used to be that we only needed to eat as much protein each day as would fit into the palms of both hands; technically, that was .8 grams of protein per kilogram of body weight per day. Newer ways of thinking, particularly as espoused for men in *The Testosterone Advantage Plan* (Lou Schuler, Simon & Schuster, 2003), pushes that amount up by 87.5 to 300 percent—meaning, particularly for guys, that significantly increased protein intake may be beneficial. These two extremes illustrate the range of opinion on the subject. We suggest you lean in the direction of more rather than less protein. Note also that protein is a strong component of the vaunted Zone and Atkins diets.

Protein also contributes to increased testosterone, which is essential to building metabolism-enhancing muscle. Testosterone is now understood to have a greater role in male weight-management functions. Schuler notes that far more studies have been conducted on estrogen, a hormone of greater importance to women, than have been done on testosterone. I concur, and present this as a further reason for guys to take a different approach to eating. And it should come as little surprise that the more active you are—and the more strenuous your activity—the more increased protein levels will improve your results.

There are differences between types of protein. Essentially, you want to eat leaner versions that come from poultry and beef, as they, along with plant sources and most fish, are better for keeping cholesterol levels in check.

As for convenience, boneless/skinless chicken breasts generally win the prize; runners-up are fancy white albacore tuna, canned beans, and low-fat yogurt. A few times a week you might take in some red meat; the lowest-fat (lowest in *saturated* fat) versions are top sirloin, top loin tenderloin, and T-bone steaks, as well as ground beef that is at least 95 percent lean (try 95-percent-lean ground turkey, too).

Additionally, innovations by the dairy industry in separating butterfat from a whipped and creamy version of whey, the protein component of milk, provide us with lots of dairy products and whey-protein concentrates that are lower in calories, fat free, and easy to eat.

A friendly, fattier exception to low-fat fish is salmon, along with other cold-water fish (including sardines, herring, cod, and mackerel). They deliver essential omega-3 fatty acids, widely regarded as healthy—and seriously absent in most American diets. Even though it may seem contrary to a weight-loss goal, certain fats, largely those from fish and plants, are considered essential to good overall health (including mental and emotional health). A complete elimination of fats from the diet is not recommended for anyone—this book steers you toward naturally finding the balance between good and bad fats.

# GOOD FATS, BAD FATS

**W**HILE THE SOURCE of fats generally helps define if they're good or bad for us, the meaning of specific fat-related terms is useful when reading food nutrition labels.

**Best Sources of Fat: Monounsaturated and polyunsaturated fats**
    Fish (cold-water fish have omega-3 fatty acids; also some saturated fats)
    Plants (avocados, nuts, corn, olives, rapeseed/canola, flax, soybeans)
**Less Desirable Sources of Fats: Saturated Fats**
    Beef
    Pork
    Chicken*
    Turkey*
    Dairy*
    Tropical plants (palm, coconut oils)
    Hydrogenated oils (usually from corn oil, a detrimental processing
        technique that creates evil trans-fatty acids)

*Most products in the saturated fats list can improve considerably when the fat is removed or reduced, such as with skim milk, low-fat yogurt and cottage cheese, and skinless chicken and turkey; certain cuts of red meat (top sirloin, top loin, tenderloin and T-bone steaks, pork) are less marbled with fat than others.

## STRATEGY #4: EXERCISE

You cannot seriously attempt to lose, gain, or even maintain weight if you don't take up an exercise program of some kind. This is only one of ten strategies, but it's half the battle. Just don't base your exercise choice on the number of calories burned during a particular activity. Tables comparing, for example, time spent in the act of weight lifting versus an equivalent period on a treadmill are misleading because they fail to take into account the 24/7 effect of exercise. The true benefit of exercises like running, and even more so with strength training, is in how such activities *build muscle.*

The more muscle you have, the higher your metabolism will be. The higher your metabolism is, the more calories you burn throughout the day. Why? Because a pound of muscle at rest burns somewhere between *twenty and fifty* calories each day, just to exist. A pound of fat (adipose tissue) will burn only *three* calories every twenty-four hours. Could the effect of strength training on weight management be clearer?

Lifting weights used to be considered inferior to aerobic activity in terms of health and weight management—but no more. In part because of this effect on metabolism, and also owing to growing recognition of the benefits of stronger muscle and bone density (you also strengthen your bones when you lift), weight training is gaining new respect. For maximum effect, don't neglect to work your legs and back because they are the body's largest muscle groups.

Some cardio activity helps round out your health. I certainly do it myself—it's as much a part of shaking off boredom and enjoying the outdoors as anything else. As an addition to weight training and smart nutrition, it prompts calorie output and a robust cardiovascular system. A Harvard Alumni Study (Paffenbarger, Lee, and Hsieh, *Journal of the American Medical Association*, 1995) found that vigorous exercise (such as swimming, cycling, and running) is associated with a 25 percent lower death rate than sedentary and nonvigorous activities (such as bowling and golf).

Working out has additional health and aesthetic benefits. A 2000 University of Florida study (Vincent, Braith, and Lowenthal) found that weight lifting protects the body against damage from free radicals, the naturally occurring, highly reactive molecules that are linked to cardiac problems and aging-related disorders such as stroke and even cancer. Advocates of free-radical reduction to prevent aging skin (*The Perricone Prescription*, Nicholas Perricone, M.D., HarperResource, 2002) also prescribe exercise as a means to achieve that result.

So reduce the calories in, increase your muscle mass (thus increasing the calories out), and you've got yourself a winning formula.

What would *not* work is dieting to the point of weakness while pursuing an exercise program. If you're weak and so don't feel like working out, it will lead to muscle atrophy, which then diminishes your ability to burn calories. Because diets are often restrictive and uninteresting, you'll go back to higher-calorie foods even while your metabolism is depressed—leading to a net weight gain. This is the "yo-yo effect"—when people lose a significant amount of weight only to regain it all back and then some.

Current trends in health-club membership indicate that a lot of men are holding up the exercise end of the weight-management deal. Men constitute slightly less than half (48 percent) of people who belong to some fitness facility (source: IHRSA/American Sports Data Health Club Trend Report 2001). The total number (15.2 million men) is up 71 percent since 1987. And for those of us who have a gym membership, we use it more often than before: 88.6 days per year, an 18.4-percent increase in the past 15 years. We hardly have an excuse not to: There are now 17,800 health club locations in the United States.

# THE ROLE OF GENETICS IN WEIGHT AND DISEASE

IT'S NOT REALLY fair, but we can blame some characteristics of our health on our parents. The findings from genetic research and the observations of genetic counselors and family-practice doctors all show how conditions, diseases, and body types (endomorph, ectomorph, mesomorph, etc.) are set in our DNA. To what degree does that affect us, and how much of a role can better eating play in influencing it?

"Twin studies have demonstrated that twins separated at birth and raised apart tend to have very similar body weights decades later," says Kristen Beck, M.A., G.C., a genetic counselor who is a member of the National Society of Genetic Counselors. "[But] when it comes to body weight, genetics does not have to be destiny in the same way that a genetic predisposition to alcoholism does not automatically create an alcoholic."

Beck notes the ongoing research into the leptin gene, which codes for a protein that has been shown to regulate body weight by inhibiting food consumption and stimulating energy use. A genetic defect that affects leptin production, while rare, can result in severe obesity. "Exercise can change your energy metabolism, and therefore you can have some control over your body weight, " she says, adding how things are much harder for individuals with this genetic predisposition to obesity.

Regarding other maladies, Beck says, "We see people who are at increased risk for cancer due to their family history and we always talk to them about methods for preventing cancer or catching it early." In addition to closer screening, some preventive drug therapies, and even surgery, genetic counselors offer patients information on lifestyle modification that includes exercise and healthier eating.

"This is true for all types of cancer," she says. "Colon cancer has been shown to be particularly responsive to dietary measures." Beck points out that deficiencies of certain vitamins and minerals (folic acid, B12, B6, niacin, vitamin C, and vitamin E)–which can result from the under-consumption of fruits and vegetables–have been shown to cause certain chromosomes to break and result in cancer. "Deficiencies of micronutrients cause cancer the same way that radiation and other chemicals cause DNA damage."

So if your mother or father taught you to eat your vegetables, they may have been trying to make up for some bad double helixes they sent your way. Be sure to thank them for that.

## STRATEGY #5: PORTION CONTROL

One reason people are getting fat is they eat too darn much. And evidence supports that. Restaurants have increased the size of menu offerings over the past several decades. The original burger, fries, and a soda at a 1950s McDonald's restaurant delivered about 590 calories; today's Quarter Pounder with Cheese, supersize fries, and supersize drink weigh in at 1,550 calories. Movie theater popcorn (buttered) used to be around 3 cups (300 calories); today, it's around 16 cups (900 calories). Economists point out that this is because actual restaurant food costs are small relative to labor, real estate, and marketing; increasing portion sizes has been a financially smart move for restaurants, movie theaters, and gas station mini-marts. Many nutrition experts believe portion sizes are a root cause of today's obesity epidemic.

The reason we eat all this stuff is probably because of our natural tendency to hoard, hearkening back to those cavemen who didn't know when the next tasty wildebeest would come within rock-throwing range. Or, in my case, because I grew up with three brothers with appetites as big as mine. At the University of Pennsylvania, behavioral research conducted by nutrition professor Barbara Rolls has demonstrated that regardless of gender, age, or body weight, people eat more when more food is put in front of them.

The solution? Eat slowly so your stomach sends the message to your brain that you're being sated. Also, given restaurants' propensity to serve bigger portions, you have further incentive to order smart when eating out (see Part IV)—it's better to eat a lot of fish and wild rice than a Fred Flintstone–size slab of ribs with fries and gravy.

The same problems can happen at home. If you make a main dish in a quantity to last three days, but then place half of it onto a big plate, you'll eat 1.5 times the calories you intended. I have done this many times myself. But just as I set my wristwatch ahead by five minutes so I can get places on time, I now use a smaller plate for my meals. It's a trick I play on myself, fully aware of the ruse. I know the portion is smaller, and I might still get up to eat a second helping (just as I might dawdle a few more minutes, knowing my watch is fast), but having to make the effort slows me down just a bit and forces me to think twice about it. A second strategy when you crave seconds is to shift your taste buds' attention to a different food. Want more chili? Eat an apple while you put the chili into the refrigerator.

## STRATEGY #6: EAT MORE THAN THREE TIMES A DAY

This may seem counterintuitive. How can more frequent eating lead to better weight management? Increase the number of eating occasions, not the total intake. Our three-meals-a-day approach is more of a social construct than a biological imperative. Whenever we eat, the process of ingestion and digestion itself expends calories. In nature, mankind ate when he (and she) came across available food. So humans got used to eating more frequently, but less at each occasion. Sit-down feasts (such as all-you-can-eat buffets) tend to put a lot of food in us at once, requiring the digestive organs to work particularly hard and rob energy and focus from the rest of the body (part of why you might feel groggy after lunch).

The fix is to snack. Snacking *smart* starts with a protein or protein/fat type of food, such as a hard-boiled egg, peanut butter (by itself or on celery or whole-wheat crackers), or a protein bar—something that will digest slowly and take an edge off your hunger. The opposite would happen with, say, a sugary candy bar or rice cake, which are quickly digested, produce an insulin reaction from the pancreas followed by post-insulin fatigue, and prompt a quick return of hunger. Better that you perform consistently throughout the day than "bonk" in the middle of an important meeting or another crunch time at work. Another smart snack is a fruit, such as an apple, pear, or orange, or a vegetable, like carrots or celery. These contain fructose, a type of sugar, but are still unprocessed carbs and as such have a lesser impact on the insulin response.

# GALLANT AND GOOFUS

**S**NACKS MAKE SENSE for a variety of reasons, but what makes a smart snack? Proteins and more complex carbohydrates, generally (but not exclusively) in the forms closest to nature, are your best bet because their slower absorption forestalls future cravings. Bad snacks are grain- or potato-based and come in a box or bag. Rule of thumb: Avoid foods that come in geometric or animal shapes.

| Better for You | Not So Smart |
| --- | --- |
| Fruit (fresh) | Goldfish crackers |
| Peanut butter | Crackers of any type (a little better if low fat) |
| Hard-boiled eggs | |
| Protein bars (if you exercise) | Chips (baked beats fried, lower in fat; but it's still simple carbs) |
| Dried fruit (limit because of excess sugar) | |
| | Full-blast sugar drinks of any kind |
| Trail mix (one handful) | Ice cream, all forms |
| Diet drinks (< five calories) | Candy of any kind |
| Yogurt (fat free, low calorie) | Cookies of any kind |
| Baby carrots with hummus | Cheez Whiz, applied directly to tongue |
| Herring (pickled in wine) | French fries |
| Nuts, seeds (one handful) | |

The beauty of snacks is that the 11 A.M. or 4 P.M. nibbles on peanut butter or apples (or peanut butter on apples) can hold you through a lunchtime or post-work workout. And when it's time for lunch or dinner, you're less likely to be famished.

## STRATEGY #7: BACK OFF FROM THE BAD STUFF

We all like stuff we know is not good for us. Things like ice cream, donuts, pizza, hamburgers, and fries. Maybe ribs, or cheesecake, or ribs followed by cheesecake. Topped with ice cream. And melted chocolate. Eating smart means facing facts without being draconian. If there is something you really, really like, just recognize that fact and realistically assess how important it is to you. Just what is it and how bad is it—is it a refined carbohydrate, or is it high in animal fat? How often do you eat this food? Can you cut that frequency in half? Can you substitute something else for it?

The great thing about having bad habits is that cutting out a few things can make a big difference. When my father was diagnosed with Type 2 diabetes in his forties, his doctor told him to lose weight. He lost twenty-five pounds in about three months by eliminating his nightly two beers with dinner (a German staple) and the evening half-can of mixed nuts, and setting limits on sugary desserts (one cookie, not four or five). He continued to enjoy each of these things for the rest of his life, but in moderation—and kept his diabetes under control through diet and minimal medication for more than twenty years.

Try shifting gradually to a substitute—for example, in restaurants ask for coleslaw or beans in place of fries. Or at least get the small portion of fries instead of the large. Eat a breakfast of oatmeal at home instead of a greasy egg-and-bacon sandwich somewhere on the road. When ordering a pizza, request half the cheese they would typically use on the entire pizza (they shouldn't mind—cheese is the most expensive ingredient). Look at anything frozen that involves a crust as a thought-starter—maybe a yen for chicken potpie means you could be just as happy with chicken soup. Reduce your consumption of anything semi-bad by half. So if you habitually eat hamburgers every Monday, Wednesday, and Friday, make the Pope and the fishermen happy by switching to fish (unbreaded) on Friday.

Learn to savor small quantities. Potato chips sold stacked in a can (you know the brand) are a good test: If you tend to eat the whole can once it's open, instead eat one chip per day, for example when you are making dinner. Take one chip only, close the can, and then let it melt in your mouth. Resist the temptation to swallow right away, just long enough to get a full appreciation for the flavor. And when you do send it down your esophagus, don't chase it with a beverage. Allow the taste to linger. Repeat this every day, one chip per day, until the can is gone. Make a bet with someone that you really can eat just one.

## STRATEGY #8: ENJOY THE WAY FOOD NATURALLY TASTES

Nature intended for us to like food. Just as with procreation, the survival of the species is ensured because mankind is drawn to the pleasure of the eating experience. For example, because strawberries taste so good, we also take in their vitamins (A and C) and phytochemicals. Nature's way is to attract us (and other mobile species) with both color and taste to, ahem, distribute their seeds. Lucky for us.

That's part of why eating unprocessed foods is almost always the better choice. Flavors naturally present in things like citrus, vegetables, herbs, and spices are strongest before processing. That's why a little bit of fat in your food—such as in olive oil, or the monounsaturated fat in nuts and avocados—is recommended. They're better-for-you fats, they make the food tasty, and they leave you feeling satisfied.

It's also why crash diets fail to work in the long run. They tend to be limited in scope, ruling out the consumption of whole categories of foods that we tend to crave. All the while the dieter wishes for that forbidden bite of bread or bowl of ice cream. The Atkins regimen pretty much rules out delicious, nutrient-rich fruits like grapes and raspberries, and tasty vegetables like corn, peas, and carrots.

Instead of focusing on living without certain things, the goal should be to stock up on great tastes you'll want to eat again and again. Strong tastes such as chili pepper and vinegar are not in and of themselves indulgent. When you free your head to start mixing things together experimentally—for example, lemon juice with a little olive oil and some spices, poured on steamed cauliflower—you open yourself up to simple taste experiences with healthier foods.

## STRATEGY #9: ACQUIRE SOME SKILLS

If you don't know how to turn on your stove, how to make a few things in a microwave, or how to stir-fry onions and chicken, you're not alone. Millions of guys don't. But that's gotta change. You'll remain a victim of the convenience-food industrial complex—and consume that average of 55 percent more calories per meal—if you relegate yourself to the unskilled.

This doesn't mean you have to take classes, purchase complicated equipment, or go to a grocery store three times a week. With the basic skills presented in Parts II and III, you can streamline the whole process so that meal preparation beats convenience food in time, money, probably taste, and certainly healthfulness.

## STRATEGY #10: DON'T LEAVE YOUR SMART EATING MIND AT HOME

You may become a great at-home cook, but you'll still eat out. It's the reality of modern life—brown-bagging a lunch is considered bad form in many workplaces, and packed schedules don't always allow for making breakfast, dinner, or snacks at home. Even though the cards are stacked against you while eating in restaurants and convenience venues (mini-grocers, fast-food drive-throughs, airports, highway oases), at business meetings, and at social events, a few tricks can help you navigate each of these situations.

So diet, schmiet—the key is to get smart, get equipped, and get to work.

# 2

# a guy's gotta be a caveman

## To rise to the next level you must first devolve

**Smart eating respects** knowledge on human evolution. Up until about 10,000 years ago, members of the species Homo sapiens ate meat (red meat, fish, and fowl) and whatever fruits and vegetables they stumbled across. They didn't depend much on grains (wheat, rice, rye, oats, hops, bulgur, etc.) because they didn't engage in agriculture until around 8000 B.C. If they chewed on a few stalks of wild rice or wheat while hiding from large-toothed predators, it still probably constituted only a tiny portion of their diets. So our bodies evolved mostly on animal-based protein and the complex carbohydrates and fiber found in fruits and vegetables (protein is also found in plant foods, to a lesser extent). When man figured out how to cultivate, store, and transport them, grains may have helped move civilization forward—but they weren't completely in tune with human physiology. (Potatoes originated in the Americas—they weren't known to European, African, and Asian populations until after Columbus.)

Fast-forward to the twentieth century, when the economics of food and population distribution—including the forces of free enterprise and a burgeoning food industry—led us to depend more on grain-based pastas, breads, rice, and potatoes. By the 1980s, "carb up" was the mantra of endurance athletes and couch potatoes alike. In moderation, that shouldn't be a problem—these forms of carbohydrates didn't poison people over the previous 9,900 years.

But modern technology turned things like wheat and potatoes into salty snacks, white breads and pastas, and French fries. When the fat-free movement went into full swing in the 1990s, food companies substituted carbohydrates (usually the simple kind, as in sugar) for fat in a broad variety of prepared foods. And everyone—dietary professionals as well as consumers—thought they were doing the smart thing by eating these foods.

The funny thing is that obesity rates went up, even more so in the past ten years. Lots of potential causes are being identified—too many fatty foods, too little exercise, dairy products, McDonald's, larger portion sizes, video games, and an increase in car commuting times. Current theories—upon which this book is based—place the blame on the endocrinological effects of eating excessive carbohydrates; the more we eat white starches (bread, rice, potatoes, and the commercial products made from them), the more our bodies are thrown into hormonal haywire. Excessive carbs actually create an echo hunger that drives further carb consumption. This helps explain why some people seem to constantly crave sugary, processed foods.

In the mid-1990s, the book *The Zone: A Dietary Road Map* (Regan Books/HarperCollins, 1995) by Dr. Barry Sears made a lot of converts to the so-called caveman diet in mainstream culture, not to mention in many sectors of medicine and allied health professions. The book hypothesizes that the evolution of mankind—starting 100,000 years ago, about 90,000 years before agriculture systems developed—came about through a diet richest in protein, fruits, and vegetables. Early humans relied much less on grains than do modern humans, and they certainly didn't have modern processing methods to alter the makeup of their foods.

The *A Guy's Gotta Eat* regimen leans in the direction of the Zone and other popular pro-protein diets (*Neanderthin: Eat Like a Caveman to Achieve a Lean, Strong, Healthy Body,* by Ray Audette, et al.; *Sugar Busters* by H. Leighton Steward, et al.; *Protein Power* by Michael and Mary Eades; and the controversial, best-selling Dr. Atkins books, *Diet Revolution* and *New Diet Revolution*). Heck, we're accused of being Neanderthals already. We might as well just go with it. According to these approaches, the heavier dependence of modern man on grain-based foods such as bread, pastas, and sugary concoctions throws our bodies out of whack. In fact, the ways contemporary humans take in most of our starchy carbohydrates—fried potatoes, white breads, chips, crackers, muffins, bagels, and white rice—were largely unknown to human physiology before the twentieth century. Early humans didn't prep for the mammoth hunt by eating penne arrabiata or cinnamon buns. Apples, mangoes, cabbage, and spicy wild chihuahuas, maybe.

Some of these authors discourage consumption of fruits and vegetables that are higher in complex-su gar content (beets and carrots among them). This doesn't take into account the multiple, beneficial micronutrients and phytochemicals that come with produce. High-carbohydrate or sugar produce is of greater concern to individuals trying to lose a lot of weight, or people who are diabetic. But for the most part, the multiple compounds found in produce have benefits that far outweigh the risk of extra calories. Weight-management professionals almost never encounter overweight people whose vice was simply too many fruits and vegetables.

If this kind of theory piques your interest, go out and buy these books. They go to great lengths explaining how this all works, with prescribed diets and recipes. *A Guy's Gotta Eat* essentially adapts the best ideas from these books to the real guy's world. You need foods you can make easy and fast. And of course you're going to eat out a lot—what you want is to know how a caveman might eat when he is in a hurry, or having dinner with a client.

# NUTRIENTS AND QUASI-NUTRIENTS, BIG AND SMALL

**Macronutrients:** The three primary categories of nutrients found in most food: proteins, carbohydrates, and fats.

**Micronutrients:** Smaller components of food, such as vitamins, minerals, and antioxidants.

**Quasi-Nutrients:** Conventional wisdom does not consider these essential to your existence, but they have significant health benefits. Fiber is a major beneficial component, but because it is not absorbed it is not considered nutritive. In addition to fiber, recent research has discovered new categories of compounds and components in the plant kingdom called phytochemicals that many qualified experts believe should be considered as important as essential nutrients. Phytochemicals are substances that plants naturally produce to protect themselves against viruses, bacteria, and fungi. They include polyphenols such as resveratrol found in grapes and wine, flavones found in olive oil, allyl sulfides in garlic and onions, lycopene in tomatoes, and sulfaforaphane in broccoli and cabbage. Approximately 900 different phytochemicals have thus been identified in fruits, vegetables, and their derivatives, such as teas. Their exact role in promoting health is unclear; however, they may help protect against some cancers, heart disease, and other chronic health conditions.

## THE NEGATIVE EFFECTS OF PROCESSED FOOD

FOSSIL RECORDS SHOW that Neo-Paleolithic humans averaged five feet ten inches in height—and to survive in harsh conditions, they possessed "the bone structures of world-class athletes," according to Sears. Since the advent of agriculture and the migration to grain-based diets about 10,000 years ago, average heights shrank about six inches. Only in the last century did greater availability of food, including more protein, enable humans to regain that lost height.

Food innovation took a turn for the worse in the latter half of the past century, when a wide spectrum of chips, crackers, pretzels, cake-like white breads, shelf-stable cream cakes, Krispy Kreme donuts, and deep-fried apple pies were introduced. Designed purely for eating pleasure with little pretense of nutritional benefit, many of these are made with hydrogenated vegetable oils, replacing beef fat previously used in commercial food production. Hydrogenation inadvertently introduced something called trans-fatty acids, which contribute to increased "bad" (LDL) cholesterol—an ironic twist, given that just a few years ago vegetable oils were trumpeted as the solution to problems associated with beef fat. Instead, we traded one problem for another. As we have moved farther away from food in its natural state, diet-related problems (such as widespread heart disease, cancers, and diabetes) have become more prevalent. Some of these factors are merely correlative; others are known to have a causative link. With ongoing research, the evidence mounts against processed foods.

# PROCESSED FOODS AND ACNE

**R**ESEARCHERS FROM THE United States and Australia are examining refined carbohydrates as a potential cause of acne. Considered a common scourge of adolescence and sometimes persisting into adulthood, acne is almost unheard-of in pockets of the world where Western-style diets rich in processed simple carbohydrates have not yet been introduced.

"There's a lot of anecdotal evidence," says Neil Mann, a nutrition researcher at RMIT University in Melbourne, Australia. Having observed an acne-free society in the Kitava Islands in Papua New Guinea, Mann is testing a low-carbohydrate diet among Westernized teenagers. "Dermatologists will tell you they have put patients on low-carbohydrate diets and seen improvements. This will be the first controlled diet."

In a similar vein, Loren Cordain and colleagues at Colorado State University are investigating the series of reactions in the body from refined carbohydrates that increase the production of acne-causing bacteria. Cordain observes that Inuit people in Alaska didn't experience acne until the arrival of the Western diet.

Look at the net result. According to USDA agricultural economist Judith Putnam (quoted in a July 2002 article in the *New York Times*), in the past thirty years Americans have increased consumption of grains by sixty pounds per person per year, and sweeteners (such as high-fructose corn syrup—sugar processed from corn) by thirty pounds. This time period coincides with the well-documented fattening of the population, and obesity rates have risen by double digits. Many people have gained weight from the colas and fries that come with our value meals, along with the chips we eat for snacks, at home and away. If we could time-travel back to the 1960s, we'd see far fewer thunder thighs in stretch pants at the strip malls. Today's hip-hop clothes are as much a functional accommodation of youthful girth as they are a fashion statement, I suspect.

## PUTTING THE ZONE DIET INTO PRACTICE

THE BASIC PRINCIPLES OF the Zone diet are fairly simple. Since hearing others talk about it a few years ago, I began to eat more beans and less rice at my favorite healthy Mexican restaurant ("healthy" because they use whole beans instead of the refried versions, lower-fat cheese, and lightly grilled chicken). I've found about a hundred ways to eat canned beans at home. I eat more chicken, tuna, turkey, and even red meat now. I experiment with lamb and pork. When in restaurants that serve it, I try the ostrich (it's not bad, and surprisingly *not* like chicken). I eat protein bars as in-between-meal snacks and right after working out (although some protein bars have more simple sugars in them than others). Protein powder is easy to put into oatmeal, smoothies, and other morning meals.

The Zone/caveman diet has its critics. As with anything, it's possible to go overboard. Many of the Zone/caveman regimen critics tell us that protein-to-carbohydrate proportions should be kept in check, and that too much meat is bad for our kidneys, livers, and colons. And they are right. Too much of anything is a bad thing. I've seen blind zealotry in some of my more obsessive-compulsive acquaintances, primarily among guys who work out a lot. What's pretty sad is when people forgo fruits and vegetables because they contain natural, unprocessed sugars (in widely varing amounts, as detailed in chapter 3). For a few calories they're shutting out the 900 or so antioxidants and phytochemicals available in plant foods. I once had a houseguest look at my refrigerator full of berries, melons, corn on the cob, and fresh peppers—bought at a farmers' market so I could be a good host—and say, "There are a lot of carbohydrates in those." He was unclear on the distinction between simple (processed) and complex carbohydrates.

Here's how you can realistically follow the Zone/caveman diet: First, try to make the pile of vegetables on your plate at least twice the size of the meat (no need to measure and count—just size it up by eye). This will help fill you up before you can overdose on protein. And for anyone concerned about a carb deficiency, note that we get simple/processed carbohydrates without a lot of conscious effort. We go to morning meetings that serve bagels, Danishes, and doughnuts. We walk down city streets and are tempted by warm pretzels as an afternoon pick-me-up. We drink beer (which has no fat, but lots of carbs). We go to ball games and eat popcorn and chips with nacho cheese, and drink more beer. In December, consultants and suppliers inundate our workplaces with chocolate-covered pretzels, candy-coated popcorn, and cookies. When working late, someone usually orders a pizza. We go to parties where everything is served on or with crackers or chips. And we love our macaroni and cheese. You will learn how to minimize your consumption of such things in later chapters. But face facts: Life throws a lot of processed carbohydrates in your direction, and it's a challenge to avoid them.

## THE ZONE OF REALITY

This approach might be called "the relaxed Zone." Basically, it allows for some starchy carbohydrates—whole-grain breads, oatmeal, wild or brown rice, sweet potatoes, spinach or wheat pastas. It's hard to enjoy a submarine sandwich without the bread, so there's no point in pretending (it makes you wish the submarine chains would offer whole-grain breads, but even their "wheat" breads are made from processed grains, though industry sources indicate they are currently developing whole-grain and low-carbohydrate breads). My big morning bowl of oatmeal includes raisins, bananas, nuts, artificial sweetener, and protein powder, and I top it off with fat-free, calorie-reduced yogurt—ultimately, too many carbohydrates for strict Zone disciples. But the oats carry great fiber and are known for various positive benefits to cardio (heart) health. With all the stuff I put in it, it's hearty and holds me until the lunch hour. And I really like how it tastes.

In a survey of fit friends, we discovered that the largest proportion of guys who work out (22 out of 51 respondents) consume some combination of oatmeal, fruit, nuts, and yogurt for breakfast (a handful of guys put eggs in their oatmeal). Second runners-up were homemade versions of smoothies—various mixtures of fruit, fruit juice, protein powder, skim or soy milk, yogurt, and egg whites, mixed up with crushed ice in a blender. Each has a high concentration of complex carbohydrates in balance with low-fat protein.

Our suggestion: Emphasize protein in the diet you control—at home, when ordering a meal, and when snacking. The easiest convenience tools are protein bars, egg substitutes mixed with orange juice, and hard-boiled eggs. Eat vegetables with your meat and beans so you fill up before overdosing on chicken breasts or lamb chops. The carbs are in the fruits and vegetables you make yourself at home; other carbs will take care of themselves outside the home.

# GOOD FATS AND OMEGA-3

IN A SIMPLER TIME, say, 1993, all the world was awash in the idea of eliminating fats from our diets. More recently, distinctions between different kinds of fats and evidence that these different fats are essential to our bodies in correct proportions have brought back some foods that are higher in fat, taste great, and are good for us. Some of the resurrected foods are high in omega-3 fatty acids, which are believed to help promote heart health, among other potential benefits.

**Sources of omega-3s include the following:**

- Cold-water fish (salmon, mackerel, sardines, tuna, herring, and anchovies)
- Wild game
- Walnuts
- Pumpkin seeds
- Soybeans and soybean products
- Leafy greens (no fat, just the omegas)
- Eggs from chickens fed omega-3–rich foods (noted on cartons)

The richest source is flaxseed oil, which can be used as a base to a salad dressing. Flaxseed itself can be sprinkled over salad, in cereal, on yogurt, or even on ice cream. Additionally, peanuts, almonds, and nuts in general are associated with a lower incidence of coronary heart disease and contain phytochemicals, believed to play a role in cancer prevention.

The fact that omega-3s are well sourced from fish fits the caveman model well. Primitive populations that thrived were clustered around bodies of water, where fish obviously are a staple.

This is not a hard routine to follow. Meat *should* be for dinner. The Zone and Dr. Atkins plans want you to include high fat along with the protein, but the average guy who eats at parties, ballparks, movie theaters, and employee functions will suffer no deficiencies of fat. If you're active and frisky, a few marbled steaks now and then make sense. I eat red meat once or twice a week. But don't take it too far—there's probably little incremental benefit in adding high-fat bacon to your burgers or your breakfast.

## PLANT MUSCLE

SO WHERE EXACTLY DO fruits and vegetables fit in? Everywhere. First, the aforementioned cavemen foraged for whatever tasted good and helped them survive. We imagine the sweetness of fruit held a lot of appeal to our knuckle-dragging and upright ancestors. I can't quite fathom how squash or brussels sprouts caught their attention, but in a pinch these probably tasted good, too.

The great news on fruits and vegetables is that scientists are finding all kinds of good things in them (such as antioxidants and phytochemicals) that they didn't know about until recently. We knew about vitamins like C already—limes and lemons helped eighteenth-century British sailors avoid scurvy and rickets while traveling for months on the open seas (hence the term "limeys"). But since the discovery of other cancer-preventing antioxidants (e.g., beta carotene, vitamin E, and the mineral selenium) and phytochemicals, we're seeing more reasons all the time to eat produce. Lately, lycopene (found primarily in cooked tomatoes and tomato products) is getting a lot of attention because it correlates with a lower incidence of prostate and other cancers. Plus, there's the fiber. If you've missed out on the fiber bandwagon and don't know what it does for you, just read the back label of a container of Metamucil. Fibrous produce and grains have the same effect but taste better. In general, a well-flushed digestive system makes sense on a lot of levels. You don't want to slow down your caveman.

Most vegetables contain some protein also, although not nearly in the concentration found in animal sources. True vegetarians have to plan their diets more carefully in order to get adequate amounts of proteins, in part because they need to eat combinations of plant foods (including legumes/beans) over the course of a day to get a full chain of amino acids, the components of complete protein. We don't want to make you have to go to all that trouble; therefore, meat eating is an assumption of this book. A few all-vegetable combinations are suggested in chapter 11, more as a taste option than as a campaign to save the baby cows.

We're told to eat as many as nine servings of produce a day—but how much is "a serving"? There's a lot of confusion on this. For vegetables, it's a half-cup cooked and a whole cup raw. For fruit it is a little bit more complicated. One small apple is a serving of fruit. But what is considered a small, medium, or large apple? For strawberries it is half a cup. But what about blueberries and raspberries? And how about watermelon? Employing water-replacement measurement technology together with coursework in calculus, we could probably figure it out. Measuring and enumerating is more work than most of us are willing to endure. So let's be beautiful in our simplicity. One banana is two servings, a larger apple is also two, and a whole grapefruit is also two. Smaller fruit like plums and small tomatoes are one serving. And it would be hard to go wrong eating *more* than nine servings a day.

Packaged frozen produce is easier to measure because the Nutrition Facts label provides portion sizes in black and white. A bag of broccoli is usually 3.5 servings. Very cool—you can cover more than a third of the daily goal of produce with a bag of broccoli as part of your dinner. Some nights it's a whole dinner, with a can of garbanzo beans, a little Caesar dressing, and Parmesan cheese sprinkled on top.

OK, so there's a little counting in that. Once you get it down, however, you'll just know you're doing the right thing by eating fruits and vegetables. Note also that you will not hear me use the term "veggies." It's not a guy word. I can't bear to say it, and I suggest you don't either. "Vegetables" and "produce" (accent on the first syllable) are far better terms for the self-respecting guy. The cutesy term "veggie" is an indicator of how food has been feminized. It's time to take back the plate, guys.

Vegetables and fruits are great guy-on-the-go food. Eat an apple when leaving the house. A banana can hang out in your gym bag all day and be protected by its peel (stick it in your gym shoes for added protection, unless you have serious fungal issues). Blueberries and raspberries are great snacks and desserts, and studies suggest that deeply colored berries are disease preventers in addition to possibly mitigating the mental decline that comes with aging. Broccoli generally requires a sit-down meal, but those baby carrots, already washed and peeled in little bags, are another food you can grab and eat on the go. On your next road trip put a bag of carrots next to your seat, just to see what happens.

The point is that while it may be technically possible, you will never overdose on fruits and vegetables. Produce, therefore, is the food you can eat anytime you please. *Anytime, as much as you want.* And feel free to do it with mustard, horseradish, hot sauce, and steak sauce (high-fat salad dressings mitigate the benefits somewhat, so instead consider lower-fat dressings).

# HORMONAL MEAT, CHEMICAL CARROTS, DOPEY FISH

**P**ROTEIN AND PRODUCE have a potential dark side. Earnest, well-meaning people rail against the dangers of hormone-injected cattle, chickens that live their short, brutish lives in tiny cages, and all those possibly carcinogenic pesticides on fruits and vegetables. And then there's the problem with additives in farm-raised salmon and other fish living in pens or "factory" ponds. My heart goes out to the chickens—even though I personally devour two to three a week. My mother tells me the poultry that her father raised tasted much better. Saturday after-noons were a wacky laugh riot in their pre-television home life when Grampa would behead Sunday's dinner; the darn thing actually ran around a bit while its cluckless head twitched on the chopping block. I'm sure our food would be better if raised in our backyards or caught while fishing. But a good chunk of Americans don't have a backyard, and those who do might run into zoning difficulties if they built a henhouse and adopted a couple of head of cattle. The "natural" versions of meats are expensive and hard to find. Realistically, factory-farm versions are all we have to work with for now.

As for the fruits and vegetables, most of the pesticides, herbicides, and other chemicals are washed off before being frozen (with a few exceptions). When you buy fresh, always run some water over the pro-duce. I put smaller stuff (e.g., grapes) in a big glass jar, fill it halfway with water, swish it around, then rinse and repeat. It's the best you can do.

## GUYS ASK WHY

**Q.** OK, so how should all of this affect my food choices?

**A.** When in restaurants, convenience stores, and grocery stores, ask yourself, "What Would Og Eat?" (WWOE). Anything in a box or a bag is suspect. Anything in its natural skin is a little closer to how it grew in nature.

But whole-wheat breads are an exception—just look for "whole wheat" or "whole grain" on the label instead of "enriched flour," which means "not whole wheat."

**Q.** Life spans of primitive populations were shorter than ours— people are living longer today than ever before. Why should we try to mimic cavemen?

**A.** Average life expectancy and life spans are two different things. It might be hard to prove the nine-hundred-year life of the biblical Methuselah, but the records show famous pre-twentieth century individuals (Hippocrates, Sophocles, and Michelangelo) who lived into their eighties and nineties. The *averages* were pulled down by killer childhood diseases and poor medical attention; those who survived were probably genetically most fit, and were just lucky enough to not have gotten kicked by horses, smitten by marauding hordes, wiped out by plague, or inundated with forty days and nights of rain.

Recent research published in the journal *Nature* ("Small molecule activators of sirtuins extend *Saccharomyces cerevisiae* lifespan," David Sinclair, et al., Harvard Medical School and BIOMOL Research Laboratories, 2003) suggests that eating certain plant foods—compounds in grape juice, red wine, and olive oil in particular—extends the quality of life as much as life span. "When you increase life span, you stretch out the entire *health* life span," said biologist David Finkelstein of the National Institute on Aging, which helped fund the research. "It's not like you're adding it to the very end to prolong feebleness."

The combination of modern medicine and food technologies make this the healthiest time ever to be a human. Make the right food choices and the *quality* of your life is improved even more.

**Q.** If the idea is to go back to nature, should we even cook food at all?

**A.** There is a school of thought (among a strain of vegetarians) that says you should eat everything raw. This offers two problems: some things taste really awful uncooked, and eating raw food allows the small critters (bacteria, tiny insects) inhabiting your food to continue living, sometimes even after your last chew. Also, you need protein, and whether it's red meat, chicken, turkey, eggs, fish, or dairy, those foods with the most protein require heat to kill the germs (with the exception of sushi and steak tartare, which are served raw). People into the raw-food movement therefore have serious limits on their options. It's true that *over*cooking hurts the nutrients in fruits and vegetables. Steaming is preferred to boiling because many nutrients leach into the water—a problem if you pour the water down the drain. But some things actually improve nutritionally through cooking and other food processing. Fat is commonly extracted from dairy, and tomatoes deliver cancer-preventing lycopene when cooked. If you're more likely to eat something because of processing—whole-grain bread versus raw grain, or frozen berries out of season—far better *that* than to eat Cheez-Its or something worse.

# 3

# a guy's gotta play in the ballpark

## The math of nutrition

**As a warm-up** to this chapter, think about the last conversation you had with your buddies about calories. Think hard. Haven't since, uh . . . *ever*? That's because guys don't talk about calories much. We rarely even talk about food except when we're hungry. It's just the way things are. You probably don't think about your kitchen as a pharmacy or biology lab. You don't want to measure and weigh or keep records. Making a meal should not be like choosing a mutual fund. And that's OK. You just have to play in the ballpark. That is, you should have a general sense about how some foods work for you, and some work against you. For most of us, smart eating is more of a *leaning* than an accounting.

The funny thing about numbers, however, is the story they tell. For example, it may seem counterintuitive to eat a fatty snack. But when you know how digestion works you can see how a spoonful of peanut butter with its slow-digesting healthier fats can ward off hunger for a few hours, helping you avoid worse snacks and perhaps fuel an hour-long workout before dinner. Some people think that beverages—soft drinks, juices, alcoholic drinks, and coffee—are inconsequential to health and body weight. They can be beneficial or detrimental; only the numbers can help you sort it out.

You could just skip this chapter. Perhaps you're a trusting sort of lad; you'll just take it at face value that the foods recommended in this book are good for you. For the most part that's true. But your knowledge will be far richer, your ability to make eating decisions much more effective, if you understand the fundamental math of food and biology, the way perpetually healthy and fit people do. They can encounter a menu in a new restaurant, or see a new item in a grocery store, and with some confidence make eating decisions that square with their overall smart eating habits.

First, let's take a trip down your esophagus and see where your last meal went.

## THE CALCULUS OF DIGESTION

THE HUMAN STOMACH IS about twelve inches long by six inches wide, shaped like the letter J, and expandable to hold about one liter of food (slightly larger than a quart), with some variance. In the case of extremely large people, the stomach can hold up to four liters (a bit more than a gallon) at a time. Solid food parks in this chamber for one to four hours— less for fluids and simple carbohydrates because they digest more quickly, longer for complex carbs, protein, and fat. About twenty minutes after filling up, your stomach sends a biological version of text messaging to your brain, saying, "I am full." During its stay in the J, food turns into a nice, usable mush (called "chyme") before being passed on to the small intestine, where most nutrient absorption occurs.

All of which gives us a few things to consider:

⊃ Your stomach space is finite, therefore so is the amount you can comfortably put into it.

⊃ The communication between your stomach and brain on fullness has a delay of about twenty minutes. If you eat fast, it's quite possible that you eat more than you need to or should.

⊃ Complex carbohydrates, proteins, and fats digest the slowest; you feel fuller longer from these than from fast-digesting simple carbohydrates (rice, white bread, pasta, candy bars, other sweets, sugared drinks).

There's practical advice we can harvest from this knowledge:

**MANAGE YOUR STOMACH SPACE:** You can eat only so much at a time, but that's a function of volume, not content. Picture a twelve-inch by six-inch hunk of cheese. You could eat it all, perhaps at a cheese-eating contest in Wisconsin. You would feel sick later, and it's enough fat to last through Lent. Do it frequently and you'll qualify to play Santa next Christmas. You could also fill up on cauliflower. Even if you ate two entire sixteen-ounce bags (frozen), it would be around 240 calories, less than one-tenth your daily requirement for calories. But that's not much fun, even if you use great spices, some Parmesan cheese, and a little butter (which might up the calories to 300 for the meal). And it wouldn't be a complete meal, more typically defined as a good mix of protein, carbohydrates, and good fats.

But if you push in the *direction* of lots of vegetables, you will create a sense of fullness before you eat too much of the fatty stuff. A quick rule of thumb is for two-thirds to three-quarters of your dinner plate to be occupied by vegetables or fruit—and that doesn't include white carbs such as potatoes or corn. The rest of your plate should be a lean protein such as chicken, roast beef, fish, or beans.

You can easily control that at home, but what about eating out? What restaurants are particularly good at is throwing white, simple carbohydrates at you—breads, French fries, and white rice, in particular. That is not good because those white carbs are way out of proportion to what your body needs. The solutions include getting vegetable substitutes, ordering items that are more meat (e.g., beef carpaccio, chicken satay, barbecue chicken) or green vegetable (salad, artichokes) than carbohydrates (quesadillas, bruschetta, corn chips). And since most meals served outside the home—not only restaurant and fast-food meals, but events such as the catered lunch brought in to work meetings—are so heavy in these simple carbohydrates, the only reasonable way to counter them is to compensate by eating far fewer simple carbohydrates at home as well as wherever possible when eating out.

## KICK-START SATIETY WITH A SLOWER-ABSORBING PROTEIN OR FAT:

Say you're feeling particularly hungry. How easy it would be to eat some chips or bread. Try something else: a handful of nuts, an ounce of cheese (cheddar, mozzarella, feta, or goat), low-fat yogurt, even a piece of herring (in wine or vinegar in a jar) or a spoonful (just one) of peanut butter. Because there are fatty proteins with distinct, lingering tastes, you get an immediate sense of gratification. Their fats are good fats, essential to the body, and they start the process of making your stomach feel like it's filling up. When you eat the main meal, you're less famished and less likely to overeat. This approach is effective both when cooking for yourself at home and when going out to a party or restaurant.

There's some evidence that highly acidic juices and foods such as vinegar or lemon juice can slow stomach emptying and carbohydrate absorption. Another plus to the herring idea. But if you're not a herring fan, a capful of vinegar or citrus alone might appeal. Or use vinaigrette dressing on greens or other vegetables before the main meal.

If you instead start out with white bread, full-blast sugar soda, or other simple carbohydrates, the opposite occurs. It's just like priming a pump—your stomach immediately absorbs these things and calls out for more. You are more likely to wolf down excessive quantities of food throughout the meal. Knowing this is particularly useful when you are around unlimited food, such as a party buffet; spend some time with the vegetable tray or grab a single handful of mixed nuts, then wait at least twenty minutes before trying anything else. There's a better chance your J-shaped stomach will send your brain the message, "Don't need that onion dip over there, it's more than I can handle right now."

So the idea of smart eating largely boils down to trade-offs and timing—the proportions of space you allocate to the foods in front of you, and eating certain foods in advance of others.

# OVERWEIGHT?
# SOMEONE HAS TO PAY THE FREIGHT

**T**HE MATH OF nutrition should include some consideration of the aggregate costs of health care resulting from bad eating. Obesity costs the United States $117 billion per year in increased health-care costs (U.S. Surgeon General David Satcher, July 16, 2002). These costs are associated with the increase in the incidence of diseases related to overeating: cancer (one-third attributed to diet), heart disease (also one-third) and diabetes (80 percent related to diet). Because costs are ultimately borne in insurance risk pools and public health-care delivery—not to mention GNP decline from productivity lost to sick days—we all ultimately share the burden, regardless of our individual health habits.

If your personal impact on the full risk pool isn't a motivator, divert your attention to a study done on 180,000 employees of General Motors Corporation by Dee W. Edington, Ph.D., researcher with the University of Michigan. Dr. Edington found that overweight and obese people in the study (40 percent and 21 percent of the total, respectively) individually incur up to $1,500 more in annual medical bills than healthy-weight people. Annual medical costs were lowest for those in the healthy-weight group.

## FOOD AND DRINK BY THE NUMBERS

### THE CALCULUS OF FOOD

Calories are a fundamental part of smart eating. They don't need to be an obsession, and there are many other things to consider, but you should have a general sense of them. What the calorie-counting system fails to factor in is the longer-term effects of micronutrients—the beneficial effects from what you're getting with those calories—as well as how different kinds of calories (protein, fat, and carbohydrates) are metabolized and used by the body. A diet that is low in calories but devoid of protein (e.g., diet soda, broccoli, and cigarettes) would lead to short-term weight loss, but would not suffice for anyone hoping to keep up muscle tone or general health. It would be effective only for losing weight in the short term, but would make the person quite unhealthy over time because a decline in muscle tone ultimately leads to a lower metabolism, which can easily result in weight *gain.*

This enlightened dietary era brings a multidimensional look at food structure. The fish you eat might be a little fattier than chicken (fats of all kinds add calories), but its good fats are essential to various body functions and overall health. In other words, don't make calorie reduction a singular goal. But the calories-in, calories-out formula still has merit— you could eat a pile of good-for-you foods (vegetables and fruit, lean meat, whole grains, low-fat dairy) and still gain unwanted weight if you're eating them in excess.

If you're interested in losing weight based on calories, start by establishing a benchmark by recording your caloric intake over a few days' time, at least as far as you can determine from food labels and what restaurants make available. For reference, depending on your body composition and level of physical activity, your daily needs are between 2000 and 4000 calories. Here's a general gauge for estimating where your needs fall:

| ACTIVITY LEVEL | DAILY CALORIC INTAKE |
|---|---|
| Sedentary/light exercise | 2000–2200 |
| (e.g., occasional short walks) | |
| Moderate exercise | 2200–2500 |
| (30 minutes cardio or lifting 3 days/week, or some physical labor) | |
| Rigorous and regular exercise | 2500–3000 |
| (60 minutes 5–7 days/week, or significantly strenuous work) | |
| Athlete | 3000–4000 |
| (more than 60 minutes of rigorous exercise 5–7 days/week) | |

Other, less mathematical ways of checking caloric input are to ask yourself some simple questions: After eating, do you feel too full? Are you on the verge of a burp in the last bite of your burrito? Those are pretty clear

messages that you ate too much. When you eat more slowly (highly recommended by food and nutrition professionals), you get the aforementioned stomach-to-brain instant message ("I'm full, please stop eating")
sooner, and you will consequently eat less.

Note that some guys are counters, people who like to keep track of
things. I think this is an influence of the information age, a side effect
of having so much of life reduced to Excel spreadsheets. I have an
architect friend who has very sophisticated knowledge of his food's
nutritional content. I will ask him, "Bob, how much fat, protein, and
calories are in that meal there?" and he'll pop off his calculation in seconds. Bob, in his late fifties and remarkably fit, also knows how much
he should eat within any day and has a mental tally going at all times.
It's advantageous but not essential to be like Bob. A general sense of
what to eat is sufficient.

The following sidebar provides the calories associated with the most
common foods eaten by guys. Think of it as your defensive game plan—
how to keep the opponent's score down. Learn to manage other dimen-
sions of food (macro- and micronutrients) and you'll have an offensive
strategy as well.

## BANANAS VERSUS PEACHES

**F**OR THE MOST part, any fruit or vegetable added to a meal is a
step in the right direction. Only if you are truly counting calories
or at least leaning toward weight loss should you pay close attention
to high- versus low-calorie fruits and vegetables. For example, you
may be indifferent as to whether a banana or a peach would taste better to you. From a calorie standpoint, there can be a big net difference: On average, a banana can have up to three times the calories
of peaches.

The caloric equation fails to note fiber and other nutritional benefits
of higher-calorie fruits such as pineapples, raisins, and carrots. But relative to weight management, calories matter. Put it in this perspective:
Deanna (collaborating dietitian on this book) has "never met anyone who
was overweight because they ate too many fruits and vegetables"—and
she should know, counseling healthclub members who are by definition
interested in shaping up.

| FOOD | CALORIES | FOOD | CALORIES |
|------|----------|------|----------|

(all in ½-cup servings, which by volume is approximately the size of a tennis ball, unless otherwise indicated)

### Best of the Bunch

| Food | Calories | Food | Calories |
|------|----------|------|----------|
| Artichokes | 40–60 | Green beans | 17–30 |
| Asparagus | 20 | Lettuce (all varieties) | 2–20 |
| Beets | 29–60 | Mushrooms | 9–44 |
| Broccoli | 45 | Onions | 10–30 |
| Cabbage | 10–20 | Peas in pods | 35–50 |
| Carrots | 25–60 | Spinach | 6–25 |
| Cauliflower | 14–30 | Sprouts | 10–20 |
| Celery | 6–25 | Turnips | 14–30 |
| Collard greens | 9–45 | Water chestnuts | 10–35 |
| Cucumbers | 7–10 | Watermelon | 25 |
| Eggplant | 11–20 | Zucchini | 9–15 |

### Middle Bunch

| Food | Calories | Food | Calories |
|------|----------|------|----------|
| Apples | 81 | Kiwi | 55–90 |
| Apricots | 40–50 | Mangoes | 54–90 |
| Blueberries | 40–90 | Oranges | 38–70 |
| Cantaloupe | 30–90 | Peaches | 37 |
| Cherries | 26–50 | Pears | 50–100 |
| Corn | 50–80 | Peas | 70 |
| Grapefruit | 34–50 | Pineapple | 30–70 |
| Grapes | 15–57 | Strawberries | 23–26 |

### Still Good for You

| Food | Calories | Food | Calories |
|------|----------|------|----------|
| Canned beans: | | Fruit preserves (one spoonful) | 18–60 |
|   Black | 100 | Peanuts | 170 |
|   Garbanzos | 100–130 | Potato (boiled, baked, or microwaved, no topping) | 120–220 |
|   Kidney | 90–130 | | |
|   Navy | 110 | | |
|   Great northern | 100–50 | Raisins | 110–130 |
|   Chili beans | 110–135 | Sweet potato | 118 |
| Bananas | 105–130 | | |
| Fruit juice blend | 90–160 | | |

### Just for Reference on Calories

| Food | Calories | Food | Calories |
|------|----------|------|----------|
| Big Mac | 560 | Corn chips | 140 |
| Supersize fries | 540 | (between five and nine chips | |
| Cola (full-blast sugar) | 360 | make a single one-ounce serving) | |

Nutritional values as provided by *The Complete Book of Food Counts* by Corinne T. Netzer.

### *Macronutrients Simplified*

Another, more complicated level of tracking your food intake is to adhere to a goal of carbohydrate/fat/protein proportions. This is where you hear various theories from assorted diet gurus: some say 40-30-30, others say 50-30-20, and Atkins and similar approaches even say 10-30-60. The numbers actually represent "percentage of calories from" the macronutrients, which therefore require adding up the grams of each item's macronutrients, then multiplying using the calorie formulas for each (nine calories per gram of fat, four calories for each gram of protein and carbohydrate). Do this for everything you eat in a day. Even better, do it over the course of several days or even weeks. Then account for your activity level; account for the amount and intensity of exercise in which you engage—and increase protein intake in direct proportion to the strenuousness of your muscle-building exercises.

Uh, sure. Do you even balance your bank statements? Don't feel guilty if you just don't feel like bothering with so much. Here's a much simpler way of going about this:

⊃ Decide where your protein proportion should fall, somewhere in the 20–35 percent range (these are skewed to the higher protein needs of men). A Zone-inspired diet will lean toward more protein rather than less, and other research on male physiology suggests doing that as well. Again, eat more protein if you work out strenuously.

⊃ Serve a meal on your plate. If you shoot for a 30-percent protein intake, subtract 10 to get 20, then make sure your protein food occupies about that much of the plate by volume. The remaining 80 percent should be produce (fruits and vegetables).

This system is imperfect and subject to variability. But if at least half your plate has vegetables on it, my bet is it's an improvement for you. It certainly is for the vast majority of adults in the Western world.

White carbs such as rice, pasta, and bread are nowhere to be found in this plan, of course; if you do choose them, you will displace the other components to your disadvantage. Exceptions are *whole-grain* versions (whole-wheat pasta, whole-wheat bread, brown or wild rice); these might compose up to 25 percent of the meal—or much less when you're striving to lose weight, replacing them with lower-calorie fruits and vegetables.

## THE SIMPLE ARITHMETIC OF DRINKS

In case you don't think of beverages as a part of smart eating, think more again. They still carry nutrients, good and bad. This includes alcohol, soda, fruit juices, "New Age" and sports drinks, coffee, tea, and water. Perhaps beverages play a bigger role in your health than you realize. Just think about it: Your morning coffee(s), your afternoon soda break, what you drink on your commute to and from work, what you imbibe at night and on weekends—these are all *habits*. Paying attention to the calories of your fluids could make a big fat difference in your waist size.

### *Alcohol*

Several brands of beer have introduced "low-carb" brews, which is a clear appeal to people now working on weight loss through a low-carbohydrate regimen. Ah, the folly. *Low-carb beer has just as many calories as light beer and only one to two fewer grams of carbohydrate as regular beer.* It's a marketing ploy, feeding off consumers' ignorance.

Light beer *is* a substantial reduction in calories for most brands—about 100 calories per bottle versus 180 or more for the regular version—so there is an advantage to going light. These vary by brand; no generalizations can be made on the calorie content of foreign versus domestic brands (check labels). Following are some numbers you can use to annoy your drinking buddies:

| ALCOHOL SOURCE | CALORIES |
|---|---|
| Regular beer (12 ounces) | 180+ |
| Light beer (12 ounces) | 100 |
| Wine (5-ounce glass) | 90 |
| | (more for sweeter, less for dry) |
| Champagne (5 ounces) | 106 |
| Spirits (1.5 ounces) | |
|     80 proof | 97 |
|     90 proof | 110 |
|     100 proof | 124 |

As a daily ritual, drinking beer and other alcoholic drinks can take a toll. If you drink one regular beer every night of every day of the year, it adds about fifteen pounds to your stomach. If you drink a light beer, it reduces that by about a third (only ten pounds gained). But most observers of party-animal behavior note that alcohol reduces inhibitions in many respects, including how and what one eats. That bowl of Ruffles with onion dip becomes mighty friendly after the second lager.

I'm not asking you to completely cut out alcohol. Prohibition failed and so might you if you create similar, absolute restrictions in your own life. Multiple health studies have shown the correlation between moderate drinking—one to two servings of alcohol per day, for example—and lower rates of heart disease, stroke, and even diabetes. The Mediterranean style of eating—vaunted for its healthfulness—incorporates moderate alcohol consumption (mostly of red wine) with slowly eaten meals, and with lower rates of disease. The key is moderation.

### Soda

Now let's shift our focus to the thing you might do all day long— drink soda. First, you have to consider the hideous nature of full-blast sugar soda. We hate to single out a particular food type (if we can call it that), but the pervasive, unlimited presence of carbonated beverages— there are 2.8 million beverage-vending machines in America—needs singular and pointed examination.

Look at the ingredients of soda. Ingredients that constitute the lion's share of the carbonated beverage industry (Coke, Pepsi, Royal Crown/RC) are almost uniformly as follows, listed in order of largest ingredient (by volume) to smallest:

⊃ Carbonated water
⊃ High-fructose corn syrup (and/or sucrose, both being simple sugar)
⊃ Color (usually caramel)
⊃ Phosphoric acid
⊃ Natural flavors (where most of the action is in brand differentiation)
⊃ Caffeine

We hope this doesn't destroy the mystique too much. It's mostly bubbly water and sugar, plus that wonderful caffeine kick. Clear sodas and even the non-carbonated "New Age" drinks are usually heavily sugared as well; therefore they offer very similar ingredient and nutritional profiles.

Now for the math. Non-diet carbonated beverages are high in calories because sugar is the only nutrient of significance in these drinks—no protein, vitamins, or other antioxidants. An eight-ounce serving of cola is 100 calories; there are eight servings in a two-liter bottle—800 calories. But a *can* of soda is actually twelve ounces, or a serving and a half—150 calories. Sit and drink four cans after lunch and you've bagged 600 calories in an afternoon. Or go get a Big Gulp at 7-Eleven for your trip home from work—800 calories.

Say what you will about artificial sweeteners, you owe it to yourself to consider the option of diet versions. They offer close to zero calories. Now, consider a switch from four cans of regular Pepsi (150 calories per can) to diet soda, shaving 600 calories off your daily intake. All other things held equal—the foods you eat, the amount of physical exercise in which you engage—look at the kind of weight reduction you might experience over time:

600 calories x 5 days x 4 weeks x 3 months = 36,000 reduced,
**10 pounds lost**

600 calories x 5 days x 4 weeks x 6 months = 72,000 reduced,
**20 pounds lost**

600 calories x 5 days x 4 weeks x 12 months = 144,000 reduced,
**41 pounds lost**

You read that right: If you switch from "regular" cola to a diet version, at four cans a day you could lose 41 pounds in a year, all other factors being equal.

# REGULAR VERSUS DIET: IS FAKE SWEETNESS INSINCERE HEALTH?

**H**ONEY WAS THE only added sweetener in ancient civilizations, but modern times have brought us so much more. Aside from cane sugar and high-fructose corn syrup—primarily used in food processing— we now have sweeteners with no calories. Much debate and a reasonable degree of concern swirls around artificial sweeteners. But the FDA has given the green light to several chemical alternatives; for anyone with a habitual sweet tooth, these provide a way to reduce calorie intake. Following the introduction of saccharine in the 1960s was aspartame (Equal/NutraSweet) in the 1980s; Splenda (sucralose, "made from sugar") and Sunett (acesulfame-potassium/K) are now approved for consumer use as well.

Some background to help you with this array of choices:

⊃ *Sugar* has fifteen calories per packet. Most sugar is ingested in processed foods (other sugars, fructose and lactose, are naturally present in fruits and milk, respectively). Excess sugar is like anything caloric: If you take in more than you expend, you gain weight in body fat.

⊃ *Saccharine* has zero calories per serving. Saccharine was the first diet product removed from the market, preceding the development of all other sweeteners. It has endured, however, in both Tab colas and the pink packets in restaurants. A lot of laboratory rats have given their lives to the study of saccharine, yet earlier warnings have been lifted because the research was considered flawed or inconclusive.

⊃ *Equal* technically has zero calories per packet. But federal labeling laws allow foods with fewer than five calories per serving to be labeled at zero. By volume, a packet of Equal has four calories in it, making it a little less than one-third as caloric as regular sugar. Individuals with phenylketoneuria, a genetic disease identified at birth for 1 in 8,000 Caucasian births in the United States (1 in 50,000 for African Americans), are to avoid ingesting aspartame because it, along with all meats with complete amino acid chains, contains phenylalanine.

➲ *Splenda* has zero calories per serving. Splenda is simple to work with because by volume it is equivalent in sweetness to sugar, enabling a simple one-for-one replacement without conversion formulas. No detrimental effects are known.

➲ *Sunett* has zero calories per serving. It is most often blended with aspartame in diet sodas, but is also available in table-top packets. No detrimental effects are known.

The biggest problem with zero- and low-calorie sweeteners is that they may provide "license" to some to overindulge in other foods. The best advice is to use them where you chronically, habitually use sugar if weight loss is a goal, but don't use them as a rationale to eat more of something else. It probably won't add up.

### "New Age" Sports and Energy Drinks

In the past ten years, the soda industry has been rocked by the introduction of "New Age" beverage brands such as Arizona, Elements, and SoBe. They're different colors, may or may not be carbonated, claim to have more adult tastes, and many boast beneficial ingredients (e.g., taurine, echinacea, ginseng) that are vaguely healthy. In most cases, the beneficial ingredient is present in trace quantities of negligible value.

Diet versions exist, but most non-diet selections list high-fructose corn syrup or an equivalent as a top ingredient. Calories per serving are around 100 to 180.

➲ *Sports drinks*—Gatorade, Powerade, and others—have a generation of sales success fueled by association with sports conditioning. From its early lime-lemon flavor to dozens more, these are not only preferred by athletes but by anyone working hard in the hot sun. The degree of benefit in these drinks is subject to dispute—their electrolytes (potassium, sodium, and phosphorus) play a role in preventing dehydration, but simple water would do the same under most moderate exercise conditions. A fair argument is that the taste drives greater consumption of fluid. Gatorade and Powerade contain about fifty to sixty calories per eight-ounce serving. Two servings per day—perhaps as part of an exercise ritual—is hardly detrimental. But if you're a sedentary person, why bother? It would be smarter to hydrate with water.

⊃ *Energy drinks* have migrated from the rave party circuit to your health club, grocery store, and convenience store in bullet-style cans with names like Red Bull, Energy Pro, SoBe Adrenaline Rush, and No Fear. You have to give them credit for truth in serving sizes: these eight-ounce cans are a single serve, so their nutritional label is at least more honest (120 calories). A diet version is about ten calories. The full-sugar versions are made up of water, high-fructose corn syrup, and small amounts of the sexy zingers ginseng, ginkgo, guarana, and taurine. Most have caffeine, which is probably the greater source of their pep.

### Fruit and Vegetable Juice

If fruit is good for us, shouldn't fruit juice be equally good? Well, close. Juices have most of the fiber of the fruit removed; even orange juice with pulp has only a fraction of the fiber of a whole orange. Apple juice is a mere shadow of its tree-born self, with skin and pectin left behind in the processing plant. On the other hand, tomato juice in particular holds its antioxidants because lycopene in tomatoes becomes more biologically available as a result of heat in processing. Antioxidants are also present in grape, apple, and citrus (orange and grapefruit) juices.

When drinking a fruit-based beverage, it is important to check the label: A "juice drink" is about 10 percent juice, much more water and sugar (identified as filtered grape juice or high-fructose corn syrup).

The bottom line is that fruit juice is high in calories and sugar; it's better to eat real fruit.

| THE CALORIES OF JUICE (EIGHT-OUNCE SERVINGS): | |
|---|---|
| V8 juice: | 50 |
| Apple juice: | 120 |
| Cranberry juice: | 140 |
| Mixed-berry juices: | 120–130 |
| Grape juice: | 160 |

### Coffee and Tea

The jury is still out on the risk/reward of coffee. Johns Hopkins researchers found that eliminating caffeine from the diet is noticeably beneficial to people with high blood pressure. Other research shows an association between coffee consumption and relief of moderate asthma, reduced depression and anxiety, and a lower incidence of kidney stones and colorectal cancers. Increased alertness and vigor from caffeine are well understood. Some research even indicates the presence of antioxidants in coffee beans after roasting; however, the degree of benefit from that is yet to be determined.

Let me fess up on this. I drink a lot of coffee. I love the smell, I enjoy the taste, and I like the way it gets me going. But I've also forced myself to start drinking tea, both green and black varieties. Its natural bitterness didn't immediately appeal to me, but the research on green tea's benefits is mounting. Green tea seems to be associated with reduced mouth and throat cancers, particularly those of the esophagus that are more prevalent in people with acid reflux (heartburn) conditions. The tannins, flavonoids, and antioxidants in green tea are believed to be beneficial to healthy teeth and gums. Over time, I learned to like it with the help of a little lime juice; I also seem to have acquired a taste for it without anything added.

But let's talk about the calories and fat that come in a cup. Without cream or sugar, coffee and tea are calorie-free. The calories you add with creamer or sugar can be significant, however; look at some of the brands of iced coffees and teas sold in stores for perspective:

- ⊃ *Venti Coffee Frappuccino (Starbucks):* 405 calories, 5.5 grams of fat
- ⊃ *Grande Tazoberry and Cream (Starbucks):* 500 calories, 23 grams of fat
- ⊃ *Grande Mocha with whipped cream (Starbucks):* 420 calories, 23 grams of fat
- ⊃ *Frozen Mocha Blast (Au Bon Pain):* 480 calories, 4 grams of fat
- ⊃ *Medium Vanilla Bean Coolatta (Dunkin' Donuts):* 660 calories, 25.5 grams of fat. (For perspective: An apple-crumb donut has half the calories and 40 percent of the fat.)

As for canned iced teas, the diet versions are calorie-free. But those with sugar have one hundred calories per serving, two hundred for most sixteen-ounce bottles. The beneficial effects of brewed tea decline in the powdering and canning process; more research is in the works, according to the Lipton Company consumer help desk.

### Milk and Whey Protein-Based Drinks

Milk is another beverage that has defied its detractors. OK, so we're the only species that drinks milk from other animals, and well past infancy at that. We're also the only primates who have figured out how to strain squash, freeze strawberries, and pound shots of Jagermeister.

I don't drink a lot of milk, but I love yogurt, and Parmesan and cottage cheeses. The beauty of milk is in the whey protein and calcium, which complement other foods in the diet and are particularly useful to guys who work out. Without going into all the science, the amino acids in whey are rich and plentiful, often sold as expensive supplements (glutamine, arginine, and lysine, for example) in dry form. Whey protein also constitutes the protein in many sports drinks and protein bars.

From a calories and fat standpoint, different forms of liquid milk vary widely (all numbers in eight-ounce servings):

⊃ *Chocolate milk:* 160 calories, 9 grams of fat, 6 grams of protein
⊃ *Whole milk:* 150 calories, 8 grams of fat, 8 grams of protein
⊃ *Part-skim (2%) milk:* 120 calories, 5 grams of fat, 8 grams of protein
⊃ *Skim milk:* 90 calories, 0 grams of fat, 8 grams of protein

Skim milk clearly is a winner with no fat and 53 percent of the calories of whole milk. Another plus of skim milk is that it has the protein and other nutrients of whole milk, as well as its many beneficial effects. Low-fat dairy in all forms is recommended for strong bones and muscles, and even plays a complementary role in weight and blood-pressure maintenance.

### Water and "New Water"

When Perrier introduced its waters in the U.S. market in the 1970s, the skeptics scoffed. They continued to scoff at Evian, Poland Springs, and the rest. Somehow, we seem to have adapted to paying for something that is usually free.

Drink up, as much as you wish. It's hard to go wrong with water. But the marketing savants have been working overtime to bring us something new: enhanced water. Think of this as an extension of the "New Age" beverages—vitamins, minerals, and a little bit of sugar in brands that include Propel, Reebok, Glaceau, Aquafina Essentials, Dasani Nutriwater, and Snapple Fruit Waters. Enhanced waters generated $245 million in sales in 2002, a 206 percent jump from 2001.

Check their nutrition labels: Some brands of enhanced water have zero calories, some as many as 125 calories per bottle; note that a 20-ounce bottle might hold 2.5 servings. The nutritional benefit varies by brand; eat an apple and a banana and you'd get more vitamins and minerals than what you might get from several bottles of enhanced water. If you drink these as a replacement for a full-blast sugar soda to reduce calories, that is a smart move, but don't expect these waters to replace real fruits and vegetables.

## MEAL ECONOMICS

NOW LET'S PUT ALL this information together into a meal. Following is a review of the calorie and protein trade-offs of smart meals (breakfast, lunch, and dinner) versus those that are commonly available in restaurants or frozen dinners. Please note, the actual quantities of foods and their nutrients that you require will vary by your body size and level of activity; the numbers here are used for a reference point. Also, the simple math of beverages is constant whether you drink at home or away, so that component of meals is not in these calculations (you can do the math yourself).

### BREAKFAST

This is the meal you should be able to control the most. Most people wake up mere steps away from their own kitchens, it's a relatively uncomplicated meal and therefore can be made in about five minutes, and consumer research indicates that morning is a time when most people have the best intentions about doing healthy things. So why do people commit so commonly the three most egregious nutritional acts in the morning? They skip breakfast altogether, they eat a muffin, or they get a drive-through egg sandwich with greasy fried potatoes. If you're asking yourself the same question about your own behaviors, I bet your rationale is that you don't have time to make something at home. Tsk tsk. Bad excuse. Let's get a little perspective:

| ITEM | CALORIES | PROTEIN (GRAMS) | FAT (GRAMS) |
|---|---|---|---|
| **Made at home** | | | |
| Oatmeal (one cup with one fruit, two dollops of yogurt, one large spoonful of protein supplement) | approx. 500 | 37 | 6 |
| Two eggs, whole-wheat toast (two slices) | 450 | 26.6 | 16 |
| Protein shake (one fruit, one cup of skim milk, crushed ice, one large spoonful of protein powder) | 250 | 32 | 0–5 |

Directions provided in chapter 11 show you how to make each of these in under five minutes, simultaneously with a shower, in many instances.

| ITEM | CALORIES | PROTEIN (GRAMS) | FAT (GRAMS) |
|---|---|---|---|
| **Eaten out** | | | |
| Sausage Egg McMuffin and home fries | 580 | 21 | 28 |
| McDonald's low-fat apple bran muffin | 300 | 6 | 3 |
| Bagel with cream cheese (two large spoonfuls) | 400–500 | 12–15 | 10–20 |

And why do we include protein content in these comparisons? You should begin to develop a sense of how much protein is present in a food relative to fat and calories overall—it's the bang for your buck, so to speak. In general, a simple way to accomplish this is to look at the Nutrition Facts label on packaged foods in order to determine if the food item of interest provides at least three times as much protein as fat. Or that the number of calories from protein (four calories per gram of protein) is about 25-35 percent of the total number of calories. For example, the oatmeal breakfast is about 30 percent (37g protein x 4 calories per gram/500 estimated calories), the eggs with toast is around 24 percent (26.6g of protein x 4 calories per gram/450 total estimated calories), the protein shake is about 51 percent (32g of protein x 4 calories per gram/250 total calories), while the McMuffin is only about 15 percent (26.6g of protein x 4 calories per gram/580 total calories).

Want to drop five pounds in the next six months? Cut out the McBreakfasts and substitute with a 250-calorie version of a protein shake (e.g., Myoplex Light) three days per week, keeping all other food and exercise constant. Directions on doing that in five minutes are provided in chapter 11.

> I always eat breakfast; it seems the easiest to do healthy: egg whites, oatmeal with raisins, bananas, and Equal. And coffee.
>
> —*Chris, San Francisco*

> Until recently I didn't eat breakfast, but now I make some sort of "breakfast sandwich," usually a multi-grain bagel or English muffin with a poached egg and turkey or soy sausage.
>
> —*Tom, Boston*

> A healthy breakfast for me consists of a bowl of [whole-grain] Cheerios with a banana and skim milk since I am unbelievably lazy in the morning.
>
> —*Tom, Palm Springs, CA*

## LUNCH

As I was writing this chapter I made myself lunch. I work out of my home, so I can do that. From where I live in Chicago, there are at least a dozen sandwich and fast-food shops and convenience stores within a ten-minute walking distance, so I clearly have options. I went to my cupboard and started grabbing things that appealed to me: a large can of tuna (solid white albacore), some new "lite" mayonnaise I decided to try, a can of black beans, a red onion, and crushed red chilies. I also took out a bag of frozen corn. I chopped and mixed everything together but the corn, which I steamed and ate on the side. Took about eight minutes to make. It was good, but I was able to finish only about 60 percent of it (the following day I supplemented it with more beans and salsa to make the concoction into a second lunch). Here's the nutritional breakdown of that meal:

| INGREDIENT | CALORIES | PROTEIN (GRAMS) | FAT (GRAMS) |
|---|---|---|---|
| Tuna (12 oz.) | 350 | 75 | 5 |
| Black beans (1½ cups) | 245 | 28 | 0 |
| Mayo "lite" (1 large spoonful) | 70 | 0 | 5 |
| Onion (one red) | 60 | 2 | 0 |
| Chilies | 0 | 0 | 0 |
| Corn (half a bag/1⅓ cup) | 200 | 7 | 2.5 |
| | | | |
| Total | 925 | 112 | 12.5 |
| 60 percent consumed: | 555 | 67.2 | 13.5 |

Now, according to an analysis of my body composition that takes into account my age (45), gender (male), height (5'10"), body weight (185 pounds), body fat percentage (variable by season, 7–12 percent), and level of exercise (rigorous and regular), my target needs are approximately:

**3000 total calories per day**
**100–160 grams of protein per day**

How do I justify so much protein? A position paper published in 2000 in the *Journal of the American Dietetic Association* (Vol. 100: 1543–1556) recommends that endurance athletes consume 1.2 to 1.4 grams of protein per kilogram of body weight (1 kilogram equals 2.2 pounds), and 1.6 to 1.7 grams for resistance and strength-trained athletes. This is as compared to the 0.80 grams per kilogram of body weight recommended for "the average person" by the U.S. Food and Nutrition Board—a clear acknowledgment that "average" can vary widely according to activity levels.

And why such a range? This, like many other aspects of dietary science, remains a debatable point. As the debate rages on, I know on a gut level what feels right to me and what I need to maintain my optimal weight and energy levels. Of course, I have regular medical check-ups to make sure my vital indicators—cholesterol and blood pressure in particular—are in check. I have no history or indicators of kidney problems, a condition that might be exacerbated by excess protein consumption. So relative to overall calories and fat grams, this one meal is within range of what I can and should eat. Still, one should look at a full day's food intake in total. Where you fail in one meal, you can make up for in another.

Had I eaten out instead, here were my potential successes and failures:

---

**MCDONALD'S BIG MAC, PLUS LARGE FRIES AND A LARGE COKE**

| Component | Calories | Protein (grams) | Fat (grams) |
|---|---|---|---|
| Sandwich | 590 | 24 | 34 |
| Fries | 540 | 8 | 26 |
| Coke (32 oz.)* | 310 | 0 | 0 |
| Total | 1440 | 32 | 60 |

*Normally, I wouldn't get the Coke, but it is cheaper as a value meal package. Of course, the diet Coke would be zero calories, shaving the total calories down to 1130, a 22-percent calorie reduction.

---

This delivers half my caloric needs for the day, is high in fat, and at best a third of what I should be getting in protein.

---

**SUBWAY SANDWICH (FOOT-LONG, TURKEY, WITH CHEESE AND HORSERADISH DRESSING)**

| Ingredient | Calories | Protein (grams) | Fat (grams) |
|---|---|---|---|
| Sandwich* | 508 | 32 | 7 |
| Sauce | 284 | 0 | 26 |
| Cheese (American) | 82 | 4 | 7 |
| Total | 874 | 36 | 40 |

*Includes bread, turkey, and "standard vegetables" (lettuce, tomato, onions, green peppers, and a selection of hot peppers), the nutrient value of which is not accounted for here.

---

I eat regularly at Subway—about once a week, a bit less than that guy Jared. But I also recognize that if I cut back on horseradish sauce—essentially made of mayo and with a portion size at the discretion of the sandwich artist—I could do better. They do offer a light mayonnaise that has only 5 grams of fat and 46 calories; if I added my own horseradish to that, it would probably taste great. In fairness to McDonald's, this meal does not include a full-blast sugar cola, which would add 310 calories.

**BOSTON MARKET**

| Component | Calories | Protein (grams) | Fat (grams) |
|---|---|---|---|
| ¼ Chicken (white meat, no skin or wing) | 170 | 33 | 4 |
| Potatoes (mashed w/gravy) | 210 | 4 | 10 |
| Green beans | 35 | 2 | 1 |
| Soda (Coke, 16 oz.) | 194 | 0 | 0 |
| Total | 609 | 39 | 16 |

**TACO FRESCO***

| Component | Calories | Protein (grams) | Fat (grams) |
|---|---|---|---|
| Burrito ("healthy chicken" version, no rice) | 227 | 25 (est.) | 8 |
| Beans on the side | 110 | 7 | 1 |
| Soda (Coke, 16 oz.) | 194 | 0 | 0 |
| Total | 511 | 31 | 9 |

*A Chicago-area chain serving "health-Mex" foods, offering the option of black beans over refried beans. Nation's Restaurant News reports that a handful of regional chains, plus McDonald's-owned Chipotle in national distribution, offer fare in this moderately growing category.

A taste favorite, this is a very good nutritional profile, in particular the protein-to-fat ratio. I often get the grande size, for which nutritional information is not available, but I estimate that ups the numbers by about 20 percent.

**LEAN CUISINE**

| Component | Calories | Protein (grams) | Fat (grams) |
|---|---|---|---|
| Herb Roasted Chicken | 200 | 17 | 3.5 |
| (Chicken in sauce, potatoes, and two vegetables—eight ounces in total, sixteen for two)* | | | |
| Total (x2)** | 400 | 34 | 7 |

*According to Nestle USA, which makes Lean Cuisine, they don't provide nutritional specifics by item because the product is measured whole as a blended mush. That works perfectly fine for me, since that's exactly what my body processes when I eat it.

** I would need to eat two of these meals to be minimally satisfied, therefore doubling the nutritional content.

Those are some trade-offs I can make in any given week. Because I exercise, I am able to occasionally eat a Big Mac, or stuff myself with the better part of a tuna salad I make at home. To keep it interesting, I rarely do the same thing two days in a row, other than to extend leftovers with a new ingredient.

The beauty of at-home eating is that I get to eat quicker because I don't have to travel to a restaurant (a little walk is a good thing, however), and I have more control, since I choose all the ingredients. If I were trying to reduce caloric intake in my at-home meal, I could simply cut back on the mayo and use broccoli (75 calories/bag) in place of the corn (400 calories/bag).

# LIQUID LUNCH

**T**OM, A COMEDIAN/copywriter in Chicago, found the lunch spots near his office to be a nutritional joke. So he started making protein smoothies in a blender at home and taking them to work in a resealable rubber container. His recipe:

- Orange juice (12 oz.)
- Kefir (⅔ cup—it's a lot like yogurt)
- Yogurt (⅔ cup)
- Wheat bran (1 large spoonful)
- Protein powder (1 large spoonful)
- Banana
- Fruit (half a cup)

*Keep in a refrigerator at work; shake before consuming.*

## DINNER

Food purveyors of all categories (convenience stores, fast food, casual dining, fancy fare) exist by a simple rule of thumb: Their food has to taste good enough to draw customers back for repeat visits. In most cases, they do this with generous use of fat, salt, sugar, and other processed carbohydrates—an easy means of creating appeal. Bread, potatoes, rice, and pasta factor heavily at most places. Did you ever wonder why the bread is free? It's cheap, it fills you up, and it goes great with drinks (where most restaurants make a sizable profit). Some establishments and chains manage to do well with healthier ingredients and menu items, but the taste experience is what makes or breaks most restaurants. In contrast, most people deride the idea of health-food restaurants—an irony, given the fact that the health club industry has more locations and members than ever before.

The Food and Drug Administration says that fine and casual dining restaurants are not required to provide nutritional information on menu items unless they make a health claim, such as "light dessert" or "heart healthy." Consequently, such claims are rarely made outside of the fast-food chains, which are required to provide such information. But nutritional information can be found for the national chain sit-down restaurants, itemized below. These give us some sense of the nutritional content of meals available at other sit-down restaurants, even if your restaurant choices are a little more up-market.

Realistically speaking, many people have less control over whether or not to eat dinner out. Dining out is a time for dates, business, or just getting together with friends. But when dinner out results from a reluctance to cooking at home, you aren't trying hard enough. The following takes a look at your options:

**AT HOME: CHICKEN WITH PEAS/TOMATOES, PEANUT BUTTER/YOGURT DESSERT**

| Component | Calories | Protein (grams) | Fat (grams) |
|---|---|---|---|
| Chicken (one breast, boneless skinless, 4.3 ounces) | 140 | 32 | 1.5 |
| Onion | 30 | 1 | 0 |
| Peas (½ box, 5 ounces) | 125 | 9 | 1 |
| Stewed tomatoes (15-ounce can) | 105 | 3.5 | 0 |
| Yogurt/peanut butter* | 160 | 8 | 8 |
| Total | 560 | 53.5 | 10.5 |

* About one large spoonful of peanut butter dipped 4–6 times into a tub of low-fat yogurt. Quantity and nutritional content are approximations.

Now let's check some comparable restaurant meals at major "family casual" national chain restaurants. These are "comfort meals," the kinds of food your mom might have made (but probably with more fat and salt, and larger portion sizes):

**SHONEY'S: SHRIMPER'S FEAST**

| Component | Calories | Protein (grams) | Fat (grams) |
|---|---|---|---|
| Shrimp dinner | 1032 | 39 | 39 |
| Cherry NutraSweet pie | 467 | 6 | 18 |
| Total | 1499 | 45 | 57 |

Shrimp can be a low-fat meal, but this version includes a lot of fattier components.

**DENNY'S: GRILLED CHICKEN DINNER**

| Component | Calories | Protein (grams) | Fat (grams) |
|---|---|---|---|
| Chicken (approx. 3.5 ounces grilled) | 130 | 24 | 4 |
| Baked potato/sour cream | 311 | 1 | 14 |
| Peas in butter | 100 | 2 | 2 |
| Frozen yogurt (low-fat chocolate chip) | 110 | 4 | 2 |
| Total | 651 | 31 | 22 |

There are better and worse items on the menu—diners are offered a selection of "sides," which range from green salads (better) to fried onion rings (worse).

**FAZOLI'S: CHICKEN PARMIGIANA**

| Component | Calories | Protein (grams) | Fat (grams) |
|---|---|---|---|
| Chicken Parmigiana | 460 | 42 | 9 |
| Chef salad (w/dressing) | 260 | 15 | 21 |
| Pasta side | 600 | 19 | 26 |
| Dressing (light) | 50 | 0 | 5 |
| Total | 1370 | 76 | 61 |

A pasta side dish with just tomato sauce would not be this fattening; with cream or meat sauce, the fat and calories add up. Frankly, I avoid pasta except in really good Italian restaurants.

**EL POLLO LOCO: CHICKEN BREAST AND THREE SIDES**

| Component | Calories | Protein (grams) | Fat (grams) |
|---|---|---|---|
| Chicken | 160 | 26 | 6 |
| Corn (3" cob) | 80 | 3 | 1 |
| Black beans ("smokey") | 306 | 7 | 16 |
| Spanish rice | 130 | 2 | 3 |
| Total | 676 | 38 | 26 |

Their "smokey" black beans are clearly a fattier version of regular whole beans.

| DOMINO'S PIZZA: 14-INCH CLASSIC PIZZA, HAM TOPPING | | | |
|---|---|---|---|
| **Component** | **Calories** | **Protein (grams)** | **Fat (grams)** |
| 4 slices (½ pizza) | 1094 | 52 | 34 |
| Soda (Coke, 16 oz.) | 194 | 0 | 0 |
| Total | 1288 | 52 | 34 |

These are not apples-to-apples comparisons, but some care was taken to select meals that a guy might typically order if looking for the better nutritional offering—each restaurant offers plenty of opportunity to get fried onion rings and other, fattier options.

# RULES OF THE BALLPARK— THE EXECUTIVE SUMMARY

SO IN CASE ALL this number stuff was too tedious for you to actually read, here is the executive summary of this chapter:

- ⊃ Your stomach has only so much space. There is a limit to what you can put into it in short periods of time. Good food should crowd out the bad. To fend off hunger, snack on food that's high in protein and good fats (peanut butter, herring, eggs, yogurt, a little cheese).

- ⊃ Beverages count. A lot of beverage marketing is misleading, yet big differences in calorie counts can be achieved with a few small alterations.

- ⊃ There are time and economy considerations, so eating outside the home isn't necessarily the death of your improved food structure. The trick is to limit routine bad habits and find balance in other meals of the day.

The bottom line is that knowing the numbers can show you how smart eating does not have to involve deprivation. Even if you don't want to spend time tracking your daily food and beverage intake, a general awareness that your choices *lean* in the right direction will usually keep you in the ballpark of smart eating. Just don't make a big deal of it with the guys.

# 4

# a guy's gotta eat simple and fast

## Convenience is greatest at home, and it comes in cans, freezer bags, and a little foresight

**It's after eight** o'clock on a work night. You managed to fit in a workout at the gym after a long day at the office. You're tired and hungry. You'll just stop at the drive-through for a fast dinner. Perhaps that's your routine, four or five nights a week. You believe it's the only practical thing. You are wrong. You could eat better *and* save time by making a smarter meal at home. And cooking the food that you really want to eat can be faster than heating up a frozen meal.

Life's most essential and pleasurable things are done at home. So how come we eat more outside the home than in? *Because we've been sold on the idea that it's more convenient.* In the case of meals eaten during the workday—lunch for most people—it is impractical to go home to eat. But the guy who buys his breakfast at a drive-through or dinner in a convenience store is misled. A lot of convenience simply *isn't.* What might seem like a good use of time quite often is not.

You are already aware that fast food isn't your smartest health option. On average, you take in about 55 percent more calories in restaurant meals than at home—that's in most types of restaurants, not just in Burger Heaven, where the percentage could be substantially more. And what's there is generally lower in nutrients than what you can get at home. Nutritionally speaking, eating out is the equivalent of shaving in the car—not only is it a less enjoyable experience, but it is dangerous to your health and appearance.

You might argue that modern times get in the way of all this cooking at home. I argue instead that modern technology is your primary advantage. How? Frozen and canned foods are not only convenient but are usually *more* nutritious than fresh foods, which means that the frequency with which you shop for groceries is a function of storage space, not shelf life. Another advantage is the simplicity of home cooking. If you had to subsist on only one cooking appliance, it could easily be the microwave—for many meals, it's really all you need. The stove-top skillet is a close second. And most food preparation is pretty idiot-proof. You just open, mix, microwave or stir-fry, and eat.

Let's examine the trade-offs by learning some basic facts about long shelf-life foods. You'll not only see how home cooking can make you healthier and save time, but how it can even help you save *one million dollars.*

## THE MYTH OF CONVENIENCE

WITH THE EXCEPTION OF the meals in chapters 12 and 13, all food preparation—from the moment you open a freezer to when the first morsel meets your mouth—should take a third of the time required for a Domino's pizza delivery (forty-five minutes). Here's how it's done with a chicken dinner with tomatoes and peas, and a yogurt/peanut butter dessert:

**DINNER AT HOME**

| *Ingredient* | *Time "cost"* |
|---|---|
| Onion (chopped and stir-fried) | 1 minute to chop |
| Chicken (one frozen breast) | 10 minutes in skillet with onion (3-4 minutes less for microwave) |
| Peas (frozen, one bag) | 10 minutes in microwave with canned tomatoes (about the same amount of time steamed); done simultaneously with chicken in skillet |
| Stewed tomatoes | 7 seconds to open can, one minute in skillet with chicken |
| Yogurt/peanut butter | (no real preparation; part of eating time) |
| Total | About 11–14 minutes |

Note that each of these ingredients is either frozen, canned, or refrigerated, and thus can be bought in quantity in advance and stored at home for weeks or even months. You can make everything (except the dessert) in a single bowl or skillet, or with the vegetables steamed separately. None of these methods involve rocket science.

Now compare that to your "convenience" alternatives:

### Frozen dinner (Lean Cuisine Herb Roasted Chicken)

Conventional oven: Preheat oven five minutes, cook 25–30 minutes, let stand 1–2 minutes. **Total: 31–37 minutes**

Microwave: Cook 8.5–11.5 minutes at 50-percent power level, let stand 1–2 minutes. **Total: 9.5–12.5 minutes**. To achieve parity nutritionals with the home-cooked meal, you would need to eat two, requiring **15–18 minutes in the microwave.**

### Eating out—casual dining restaurant

Transportation: 10 minutes to get there and park

From being seated to ordering: 10 minutes

From ordering to service: 8 minutes

Eating the meal: 12–16 minutes

Eating dessert: 10 minutes

Paying the bill: 6 minutes

Transportation home: 10 minutes

**Total: 56—70 minutes**

### Eating out–fine dining restaurant

Transportation/valet parking: 20 minutes
Waiting for a table: 0–60 minutes
From being seated to ordering: 15 minutes
From ordering until food arrives: 20 minutes
Eating time: 30–90 minutes
Paying the bill: 8–12 minutes
Waiting for the car from the valet: 2 minutes
Transportation home: 20 minutes
**Total: 100–224 minutes**

### Take-out–phone-in

Time spent looking for and perusing menus: 10 minutes
Time on the phone to order: 5 minutes
Transportation to restaurant: 5 minutes
Paying for food: 3 minutes
Trip home: 5 minutes
**Total: 28 minutes**

### Delivery–phone-in

Time spent looking for and perusing menus: 10 minutes
Time on the phone to order: 5 minutes
Time spent on phone when they call to confirm your order: 1 minute
Waiting for delivery: 30–60 minutes
Payment transaction at the door: 1 minute
**Total: 47–77 minutes,** albeit you could be doing something produc-
tive other than watching television while waiting the 30–60 minutes
for delivery

### Drive-through–fast food

Detour from normal route home to restaurant: 5 minutes
Time waiting in line: 10–20 minutes (rush hour)
Transaction at drive-through window: 3 minutes
Eating: 2 minutes
Driving home: 5 minutes
**Total: 23–33 minutes**

If you're skeptical about how much time at-home cooking takes,
you're being reasonable. Chances are, you will take a few extra minutes

the first few times you try it. But note also the "Five Minute Wonders" in chapter 11, which beat all of these "convenience" approaches hands-down.

## STOCK UP ON GROCERIES

AND WHAT ABOUT THE time to shop for all this food? Figure that will take you 60–90 minutes per month, probably less if you do online grocery ordering and delivery. Spread over 30 breakfasts, 8 lunches, and 16 dinners per month, you can tack on an additional 1.1 to 1.6 minutes per meal made at home.

But can you shop just once a month or less? Once again, modern technology makes it easy. Most guys seem to like the idea of minimal shopping. If you have to invest more time in this task than you are willing to give it, the whole thing falls apart. That's why the *A Guy's Gotta Eat* plan requires you to shop only once a month. Actually, you can even shop less often than that.

Frozen vegetables, canned beans and tomatoes, and foods that keep for weeks in refrigerators (yogurt, cottage cheese) are the basic staples you can keep around the house for any time you need a snack or a quick meal. Frozen chicken and beef and canned tuna are also a big plus. Here are some facts about frozen, canned, and dried foods that make many of these foods smart choices:

⊃ *Nutrient retention:* Frozen and canned vegetables and legumes contain more nutrients than those sold fresh. This is because the nutrients in frozen produce are locked in through "flash freezing" within a day of harvest, while the "fresh" stuff spends as many as fourteen days on a truck, in a warehouse, and in the produce section of the grocery store before you even buy it. Air and time degrade nutrients in all fresh produce. Additionally, heat processes involved in canning (of vegetables, legumes, fish, and poultry) sometimes enhance the bio-availability of certain nutrients (e.g., lycopene in tomatoes). Canned beans have slightly better nutrient retention than those that are dried and then soaked overnight by the cook (which you wouldn't do anyway). This was studied extensively in the mid-1990s by researchers at the University of Illinois Department of Food Science and Human Nutrition (B. Klein, et al.), dispelling years of erroneous assumptions and outright disparagement of canning and freezing.

⊃ *Nutrient density:* Some versions of frozen foods actually deliver more nutrients. In the case of chopped broccoli (sold frozen only) versus broccoli spears (sold fresh and frozen), the greatest concentration of nutrients is in the bulb or head, the primary component of chopped broccoli. Ounce for ounce, chopped frozen broccoli is your best nutrient-dense buy.

⊃ *Preservatives beat the alternative:* A few decades ago people became alarmed by the presence of preservatives (BHA, BHT, dehydroacetic acid, etc.) in foods. That furor has simmered down considerably. The FDA has carefully scrutinized independent studies on the most commonly used preservatives, and formulated use criteria for manufacturers. In the meantime, public pressure has driven many manufacturers to use non-chemical methods to create shelf stability (herbs and ultraviolet light-blocking packaging, for example). Looking back into the historical archives, we should note that about eight hundred people died in the first half of the twentieth century from botulism; today there are far fewer cases, with most cases related to home canning and intravenous needle use. No body of research has established a definitive link between chemical preservatives and illness. Note that preservatives are largely *not* used in vegetable preservation—rapid-freezing technology is a physical process—nor in products that are acidic or heavily salted. Primarily, preservatives are spoilage and bacteria retardants for baked goods and other processed foods, including canned beans.

⊃ *Economics:* It's obvious that spoiled food is lost money; frozen, canned, and dried goods prevent that loss. Additionally, a study by the U.S. Department of Agriculture found that most frozen vegetables were less expensive, pound for pound, than fresh. This is partially due to the price variances of "in season" versus "off season," since frozen food is sourced at the most economical (in-season) prices.

All these benefits aside, if you heap a few portions of peas on your plate you're far ahead of the guys eating onion rings, regardless of whether your peas are frozen, canned, or fresh.

## SHOPPING ONLINE

I purchase about 90 percent of my food through the online grocery service available where I live (Peapod in the Chicago market). It's hugely practical and I usually save enough by scanning for marked-down specials to offset the modest delivery charge (around $5). It takes about twenty minutes to place an order, and another twenty minutes to receive and store items when they arrive. The downside of online grocery shopping is that I tend to browse the aisles less, instead reordering items I've purchased in the past; that's why I also visit the grocery store from time to time.

Online grocery seems to be preferred by small households. Fully 57 percent of shoppers at Peapod are from one- or two-person households.

**K**EITH OF LOS ANGELES, a busy and fit CEO, sometimes includes about one hundred pounds of bottled water with his weekly online grocery order. "[It's a] $4 delivery charge and sometimes that's waived," he says. He self-rates his at-home eating habits as "very healthy." They include smoked salmon on whole-wheat toast (for breakfast) and peanut butter sandwiches dipped in skim milk—not something this Ivy League MBA would be free to do at the office.

Here is a list of online grocers. It is subject to change at any moment, but is likely to stabilize and grow as companies find successful business models. Also, many smaller chains are starting their own proprietary services (ask at the customer service desk in your grocery store). Most charge a delivery fee of between $5 and $10, less for larger orders or if you pick up your groceries yourself (think of it as drive-through grocery shopping).

### Peapod.com

Currently serving Chicago, Washington, D.C., Boston/Cape Cod/Worcester, MA, Providence, RI, Long Island and Westchester County, NY, and Fairfield County, CT, Peapod appears to have survived its battle with defunct competitors (Webvan, Shoplink, Streamline, HomeRuns, and Priceline) since being acquired by Royal Ahold, a Dutch company that owns several grocery chains in the eastern United States

(Stop & Shop, Tops, Bi-Low, and Bruno's). Spokesperson Annette McMillan says that expansion will likely occur in markets where these stores are located; also, sales for 2002 were up 35 percent in existing markets from 2001, a trend that bodes well for further development of this new retail channel.

### Albertsons.com

Currently serving Los Angeles, Orange County, San Diego/Riverside, San Francisco, and the Bay Area, CA, Las Vegas, Portland, OR, Seattle, and Vancouver.

### FreshDirect.com

Available in portions of the greater metropolitan New York area (mostly Manhattan), industry trade publications are examining this store as a new model for online grocery success.

### Safeway.com

Backed by Tesco, the U.K. grocery giant that has established success in online grocery retailing, this established supermarket chain is effectively reaching customers in Northern California, Oregon, and Washington, and through its Vons subsidiary in San Diego County.

### Schnucks.com

This St. Louis-based retailer is an example of traditional grocery stores making headway by serving traditional customers with online ordering. Other examples are PublixDirect (south-Florida markets only), Marsh (Indianapolis), Hy-Vee (Des Moines), and D'Agostino (New York).

### NetGrocer.com

Delivers nonperishable goods nationwide (in the forty-nine continental states, not Hawaii); shipping rates are steep (10–30 percent of the value of the order).

# GETTING FRESH

**O**K, SO NOT everything that's frozen is the same as fresh. Green leafy stuff, for instance. Frozen spinach is not at all like fresh (even though the nutrient levels of frozen spinach are better). For perishable items, the once-a-month shopper will enjoy fresh goods only one week out of four. So what do you do the other three weeks? Here are your options:

- Order whatever you're out of at home when you eat out.
- Do a spot-visit to a supermarket or convenience store that carries a limited line of fresh goods every couple of weeks.
- Practice balance, variety, and moderation. If you eat fresh greens one week out of the month, make sure you eat frozen vegetables the other weeks.

The produce industry has wisely learned to cut and wash a broad variety of greens and sell them by the bag. Take advantage of this.

## WHERE YOUR MONEY GOES

SIMPLE AND FAST FOOD at home also translates into a lower price tag. Consumers, particularly younger ones, are catching on to this fact. According to the Food Marketing Institute (FMI), which represents 26,000 retail food stores, consumer purchasing data in 2002 indicates that people are making more meals at home than in the recent past. This is a reversal of a long-term trend of purchasing meals outside the home, a consumer behavior that began in the 1950s with the birth of fast food. Fully 79 percent of young adults eat out two or fewer times each week—largely due to economic factors, says FMI. In particular, younger shoppers who frequently eat meals outside the home (three or more times per week) reduced their consumption of such meals by 46 percent since 2000. Somewhat related to this is the fact that half of shoppers are "very concerned" about the nutritional content of what they eat.

In general, these are good signs. People are taking more control of their food structure, even if it is for reasons other than nutrition. For the people who are truly thinking, it's a great time to pick up smart eating skills.

Let's look at the cost of a prototypical dinner to find out how much money you will save by eating at home:

| DINNER AT HOME | |
| --- | --- |
| *Ingredient* | *Grocery cost* |
| Chicken (one breast, boneless/skinless) | $1.43 ($9.99 per 2.5-pound bag of 6–8 breasts) |
| Onion | $0.69 |
| Peas (one bag) | $1.89 |
| Stewed tomatoes (one 14.5-ounce can) | $1.25 |
| Yogurt/peanut butter | $0.93 ($0.66 + $0.27) |
| Condiments, spices, and oils | $0.25 (approx.) |
| Total | $6.44 |
| (no tipping necessary) | |

For comparison, we did a sampling of similar "home-style" restaurants—where the food ain't any fancier than what you make at home—including Shoney's, Denny's, El Pollo Loco, and Fazoli's, plus Domino's Pizza for its ubiquitousness and because it's a general default to the unimaginative eater. In general their prices (plus a 15 percent tip) came to between $10 and $14 each, even allowing that the $20 pizza can be split into two meals. On average, a regular workaday meal made at home might save you around $3.50, probably more. Do that 4 times a week, 48 weeks out of the year and you'll squeeze out $672 to spend on something more interesting.

And each of those is considered a value/economy restaurant. So let's assume you are a swanky guy who likes to be seen in snazzy places, like this month's hot new restaurant. You have the economic discretion to eat out two nights (or more) a week in stylin' bistros, where you spend an average $45 per meal (this includes a drink, appetizer, entrée, tip, and car valet, parking, or taxi). You could eat at home, but you'd rather spend a few hours with friends than be home cooking and watching *Friends*. But here's the cost over a year:

$45.00

−$6.44 (cost of making it at home)

= $38.56 incremental expense

    x 2 occasions per week

= $77.12/week

    x 48 weeks of the year (you will miss a night here and there)

= $3701.76 incremental expense per year

Some people can afford this, and, by golly, our economy needs the boost. But according to my financial planner (Joe Esposito of Esposito, Kiker & Associates in Glen Ellyn, IL), if you invest that same money in a mutual fund over the course of ten years—say, between the ages of twenty-five and thirty-five—it would accumulate at 10 percent compounded interest, the approximate average for the S&P 500, to $58,996.52. Hold it in a mutual fund with no additional contributions until you retire at age sixty-five, and you end up with $1,029,454.02 *extra* at your retirement. With that kind of money, you can take your friends to *France* for dinner.

Now go back to those nights when you are leaving the office, gym, or someplace else and are hungry. Envision how you'll get home half an hour sooner because you don't stop for greasy food somewhere. Picture how in fifteen minutes—time during which you'll cook and catch up on voice mail, turn on the TV, or talk on the phone to a friend—you'll have a high-protein, high-fiber, elevated-antioxidant meal that tastes great.

You're beginning to see yourself as a very smart guy.

# 5

# a guy's gotta respect his vices

## Smart eating doesn't have to be an all-or-nothing proposition

**Let's be honest.** There is a pizza in your future. There's even a pile or two of French fries. Maybe a McRib sandwich here and there. And some Krispy Kremes. You gotta live, and sometimes that means eating what's being served or what's available. People who tell you otherwise haven't got a clue as to what it means to be a guy living in the real world.

The place to draw the line between realistic and dangerous is when eating bad-for-you foods becomes chronic. For example, eating a bag of buttered extra-salt popcorn every time you go to the movies, or a drive-through meal two or more times a week. Or having ice cream after dinner every night. You can eat indulgent foods on special occasions. But the sobering reality is that *you* suffer when you eat these things in great quantities all the time. The shame is when a single vice sabotages your better intentions—such as how a high-carb, high-fat lunch every day wipes out the benefits of a spin class or a healthy dinner. If you consciously acknowledge your vices, respect how much you enjoy them and what damage they might do to you. From there, learn to strike a balance between healthy and unhealthy eating.

You don't have to cut out anything in its entirety *if* you can manage to maintain a low frequency and quantity. Take control. Eat crispy chicken only at outdoor picnics. Eat ribs when you go to a rib house, and no more than, say, once a month. Set your pizza limit to once a week—even better if it's a reward for keeping up a good workout schedule. This requires a mix of willpower and wits—more of the latter reduces need for the former. Learn a few tricks and you'll feel far less deprived.

# SERIOUS OVEREATING

**T**HERE IS A degree of overeating beyond the scope of this book: compulsive overeating with psychological underpinnings. Thousands if not millions of Americans overeat for reasons that go far deeper than satisfying a craving. I read testimonials on the Overeaters Anonymous Web site (http://www.oa.org/index.html) and acknowledge that such issues are serious, complex, and need focused attention.

If this book helps you break an eating addiction, great. But I encourage anyone who feels this is beyond their control—perhaps, after you attempt the advice provided in this book but fail to achieve a noticeable result—to seek professional support. The quality-of-life improvements from eating smart should be accessible to everyone.

But all of us can borrow some ideas from Overeaters Anonymous, which adheres to the same 12-step program model used by Alcoholics Anonymous and other addiction-recovery movements. Each of them espouses surrendering to a higher power and making amends with friends and family. I will suggest that adopting a smarter approach to eating, even reducing our own moderately bad habits, is about others as much as ourselves. The body is a temple, after all. We should seek maximum health for the sake of our life partners. We should be healthy if we have children. We should even be healthy for the sake of our parents, who might need assistance from us as the years wear on. With greater vitality and physical abilities come so much more, particularly a better shot at financial and physical security and emotional support for those around us.

A guy's gotta be a good friend, husband, father, and son, too.

## HOW TO DE-VICE

THE DEGREE TO WHICH you wish for change will determine how much effort you'll put into it. Are you attempting to change your appearance through weight reduction or muscle building? Are you motivated by the general sense that eating smart would improve your health as you age? Are you doing this to achieve a short-term goal, like getting ready for summer beach parties or a class reunion? Vice management is most successful when you have a clear understanding of your goals.

You might consider the following six-step approach:

**1. IDENTIFY YOUR VICES:** You should know by now what your food or beverage vices are. If they are specific foods, you might also give some thought to occasions when you eat them. Are these part of rituals, such as "after work" or "weekends" or "at parties" or "lunch near the office"? Determine how many are driven by situations and how many are a simple matter of you loving something a little too much.

Try to come up with a list—most people have a primary vice and several secondary ones. Then take a step back; a sensible approach is to tackle one or two vices at a time. Just be sure not to overcompensate by trading one vice for another.

What are the most common vices?

### That One Thing You Love

Like a bad-for-you lover, you crave the thing most forbidden to you. If the Dunkin' Donut's shop on your way in to work inspires a happy feeling inside, you know you have a monkey on your back (and a reason to change your route).

### Convenience Cuisine

It's not one food, it's a category of foods. Fast-food restaurants and even convenience stores have made some notably healthy additions to their menus and product offerings in the past couple of years; however, the bulk of sales are still of processed foods that are heavy on carbs and fat. Challenge yourself to find a better thing to eat next time you're at Burger King or McDonald's. That includes getting a beverage that is not primarily made of sugar.

### Excessive Portions in Restaurants

This is a problem in all types of restaurants, as the average portion sizes have increased across the board in recent years. And men are more susceptible to overeating when faced with large portions. A survey by the American Dietetics Association ("Nutrition and You: Trends 2002") revealed that when faced with an excess of food on a plate, men are almost five times more likely to finish it off than women (women actually consider it a social grace to leave a little bit of food on their plates—but with larger portions they, too, eat more).

### Eating at Home—Two Dinners Instead of One

They say never trust a thin chef, and I know why. When you cook at home you discover how great it can taste. You also realize it's just as easy to make four portions instead of one or two, intending to save some for later. Then you effectively eat two or three meals in one sitting. A rule of thumb is to dish up the portion you intend to eat, then put the rest away in the refrigerator. To go back for a second helping will require a few more steps than just serving another portion from the stove top—a small barrier that at least makes you think twice.

### Alcohol-Induced Indulgence

It's partially the booze itself, but it's also the loss of inhibition that matters. And where else do we typically find both in abundance than at parties? When you're drinking, you're more likely to eat six handfuls of the Chex Party Mix. Depending on the individual, a moderate amount of alcohol (thirty grams of alcohol a day, or the equivalent of three to four glasses of wine) produces a range of negative short-term effects on the body, including an increase in heart rate, heart palpitations, an increase in skin temperature, muscle weakness, and facial flushing. Alcohol also promotes water loss from the kidneys, which can lead to dehydration, particularly among people who drink spirits (which have a higher concentration of alcohol) without consuming extra water. Each of these things will tend to reduce your physical activity, which results in a lower metabolism and easier weight gain.

Looking at it from the long term, excessive alcohol consumption alters the balance of reproductive hormones, according to a collection of studies compiled by the National Institute on Alcohol Abuse and Alcoholism. In excessive cases, alcohol metabolism contributes to testicular injury and impairs testosterone synthesis and sperm production. In a study of healthy men who received 220 grams of alcohol (about sixteen drinks) daily for four weeks, testosterone levels declined after only five days and continued to fall throughout the study period. Prolonged testosterone deficiency may contribute to feminization in males (for example, breast enlargement). In addition, alcohol may interfere with normal sperm structure and movement by inhibiting the metabolism of vitamin A, which is essential for sperm development.

### Easy Ruts

We all have our rituals and habits. The beauty of predictability is how it frees our minds to concentrate on other things. The problem comes when the rituals are detrimental and degenerative over time. Breakfasts are the best example, because the things we do in the morning are generally the most ritualistic of all—guys tend to go through the motions before our brains are fully capable of decision making. If your ritual is oatmeal or a fruit/protein blender drink, chances are it's a good habit. But say you always put raisins in your oatmeal, never alternating with blueberries, strawberries, apples, or other fruit. That would tend to limit the types of vitamins, minerals, antioxidants, and fiber you consume to your body's disadvantage. The principle of balance, variety, and moderation suggests mixing it up now and then just to give your body a chance to absorb new nutrients.

**2. KNOW WHAT YOU'RE UP AGAINST:** The forces of free enterprise and marketing catch you at every turn—reportedly about one thousand advertising messages hit you every week. Here are some examples of how the purveyors of the aforementioned cheap agricultural commodities—processed grains, potatoes, and sugar—are chasing you down:

⊃ *Action-Oriented Pizza:* Pizzas have some good stuff in them (tomato sauce, vegetables, and even protein). But a spokesperson for Pizza Hut, a stress management expert at that, said in a 1998 press release: "As our lives become more hectic and stressful, the need to occasionally indulge and reward ourselves increases. A new survey reveals that today's young men (ages 18–29) choose zestier, more intensely flavored food to indulge in, similar to their adventuresome, action-oriented lifestyle that keeps them tuned in to extreme sports." So, on a stomach full of cheese, sausage, and baked dough, we're indulging in the adventure of watching TV. Impressive. That's how they think of us. Incidentally, another study also conducted in 1998 for Pizza Hut showed that men aged 18–29 ranked their favorite indulgences in this order: pizza, ice cream, steak/beef, chips, and cookies. Guys, they might understand our vices better than we do—although steak and beef can easily fit into the virtue column.

⊃ *Gridiron Gastronomy:* Ads on the Super Bowl—all sports programming skews male—are largely for high-fat, high-calorie, nutrient-poor foods. The January 2001 contest (Baltimore Ravens over the New York Giants, 34–7) featured the following at halftime: M&M/Mars' Snickers Cruncher Bar, Frito-Lay's Ruffles Flavor Rush Ruffles, Doritos' Nacho Cheesier, and full-blast-sugar Pepsi-Cola. And that's all while we're drinking beer. One hopeful note is that Subway sandwich shop's Jared, the guy who lost about half his body weight on his (healthy) submarine diet, was also featured in the game's commercials.

⊃ *Low-Rent Luxury:* And on the subject of snack foods, according to a report in *Supermarket News* (May 7, 2001), the $6 billion snack food category (includes salty, savory, bakery, "better-for-you," and sweet) grew 27 percent in the previous five years. Think about that. This is a mature industry, where growth rates in the single digits would be far more likely. They've clearly come up with new ways of getting more of us to buy and eat *significantly* more of their food. ("Better-for-you" is an industry designation for confections such as Snackwells, not necessarily a designation made by nutritionists.) Most of these items are made with processed carbohydrates; the cheap flours, potatoes, and sugars. An industry spokesperson crowed, "Snacks and chocolates are recession foods. They are that

indulgent treat that's still affordable when money gets a little tight."
Chuck that trip to Cancún, it's time for a King Size Milky Way Bar.

Of course, not everything produced by the food industry is bad. But if
you rely on advertising to get nutrition advice, you are in trouble. Chew
on these numbers: McDonald's alone spent $1.1 *billion* on advertising
worldwide in 2001; in the same year, the U.S. government's entire promo-
tional budget for the "5 a Day for Better Health" program was $1.1 *mil-
lion*. TV, billboards, and radio advertising are not working in your favor.
So what is there to learn from all this? The ability to overcome food
vice lies in your inner resolve to beat the advertisers at their own game.
Knowledge is one of your best weapons against chronic food vices.

**3. ASK YOURSELF, "CAN I LIVE WITH LESS OF THIS?":** It's important to have limits. Setting limits and adhering to them is gratifying, and
a reason to feel good about yourself. Note how it's not about abstinence.
When you play in the ballpark of smart eating, the game includes a few
pop outs on the way to scoring a few runs. This is about raising your hit-
ting stats by improving your form. Make it a commitment, then turn that
commitment into action: Quit driving on streets with donut shops or just
keep junk food out of your house.

**4. ESTABLISH A FREQUENCY OF ACCEPTABILITY:** Vice reduction is
best accomplished with the least amount of pain. So if you cut back on
something without cutting it out entirely you're less likely to feel
deprived—and therefore more likely to succeed.
For example, say you eat a bag of potato chips every week. You decide
you want to reduce this to, say, one-quarter of that. Rather than trying to
eat a quarter of the bag each week, you might just eat one bag once a
month in a single sitting. If you instead dole out the bag over four weeks,
you might rationalize that the chips will lose their crunch with time, then
eat the whole thing some dark and stormy night. It's better to restrict
your chip-eating habits to occasions when they are served at parties. But
the alternative approach might work, too. I tested myself at eating a single potato chip every evening while making dinner. Just one chip. It was
a ridiculous goal, but I managed to do it. I savored the chip for as long as
I could, appreciating it for all that it could be, and at the same time, learning to appreciate all that it was not. It taught me that I could stop at one,
and that I could experience a lot of taste with this single chip.

**5. SHIFT GEARS:** If you're like me, you love peanut butter. Or maybe it's something else that you keep around the house, such as leftovers from that great meal you just made yourself—a healthy food in moderation, but a problem when you eat too much. I'm pretty good at eating a small spoonful of peanut butter once a day, usually an hour or so before going to the gym. But sometimes it is mighty tempting to have a second spoonful. Perhaps even a third. When faced with that temptation, I try to shift my brain to another taste, usually something distinct and different. Pepperoncinis (a type of pickled peppers) are effective—spicy and vinegary, I can eat one or two of them and divert my thoughts away from peanut butter. Pickled herring works, too, as do fruits and vegetables, such as apples, pears, baby carrots, and celery. Just get off the track of that one food craving before you ride recklessly all the way to the bottom of the jar.

**6. DILUTE THE VICE:** Maybe your weakness is macaroni and cheese. You love that buttery, creamy texture and the feel of all those little slippery elbow pastas in your mouth. It's primarily a meal of processed carbs with lots of fat, but knowing that just isn't enough to stop you from making and eating it; heck, it was probably the first thing you learned how to cook. If you must have it, start mixing a bowl with a whole bag of chopped broccoli (throw it into the boiling macaronis in the last minute or two of cooking), or add kidney beans just to raise the protein level a bit.

Ice cream lovers can do something similar. Buy a single flavor (vanilla, chocolate, or whatever) without the chunky parts—things mixed in like cookie dough usually add more fat and sugar than the base ice cream. Put it in a bowl; don't eat out of the pint carton. Again, cut back a little here—a pint container is considered four portions (check the Nutrition Facts label). Now add raisins, berries, orange slices, or apple chunks to your ice cream. *Come on*, just give it a shot. Get some of those nine daily servings of produce right there at dessert time. In a few days or weeks or a year, try to move on to a new taste—fat-free vanilla yogurt—and mix in the same fruit. *Just try it.*

Don't get too hung up on your food vices, because the real point of eating smart is finding the foods that you enjoy. Done smart, you'll learn to indulge in the pleasure of good health.

# 6

# a guy's gotta eat like a guy

## Inherent advantages over girls that most guys don't know about

**It doesn't take** a genius to see that women and men are physically different. Recent scientific research has shown that the genetic gulf between men and women is bigger than previously thought. And numerous books have established how our psychological development figuratively occurs on separate planets, Venus and Mars. It should be no surprise, then, to note that how much guys eat, why we eat, and what happens when we eat is also different. So why are matters of food and nutrition almost always discussed as if we are all the same? Next time you see something in the news about nutrition, pay attention to whether they distinguish between women and men. Usually they don't.

The differences are astounding. Most encouraging is how men are imbued with distinct advantages where it comes to weight maintenance. For example, men's cravings of foods such as red meat with just a little fat might be just what nature intended for us. If we learn we have to refrain from eating certain foods, we seem to be equipped to handle that without a lot of fuss. Underlying all of this are specifically male characteristics of intellect and a sense of responsibility, each of which makes health improvement more likely.

But gentlemen, we have a problem. It appears as if men are losing in the health game—in measurable ways, more now than just fifteen years ago. And younger guys are getting fatter faster than the older guys did, despite our inborn advantages. Let's call it the Guy Paradox. The main markers of the Guy Paradox are obesity and poor weight management.

According to the U.S. Centers for Disease Control, here's what's happened:

| PERCENT OBESE BY GENDER (U.S.) | | |
|---|---|---|
| *Group* | *1991* | *2000* |
| Male | 11.7 | 20.2 |
| Female | 12.2 | 19.4 |

In a decade, we went from one in ten to two in ten guys tipping the scales to an unhealthy point. And we overtook the women—perhaps we got a little too exuberant with this gender equality thing? We seem to not be trying. Or we're not paying attention. We're not leveraging the advantages we have as guys. We seem to have lost something in modern living that defined us one hundred, one thousand, and one hundred thousand years ago. We were the stronger sex; we were designed to hunt, capture, and drag the goods back to the cave. The stronger and smarter among us survived, partly from an obligation to take care of kith and kin—but no more. Hence the paradox.

But you, bud, can get back to your ordained physical self when you unravel the mystery of what to do about it. To get you on your way we present a dozen reasons why and how guys can succeed at smarter eating (no girls allowed!).

**1. RESPONSIBLE GUYS EAT SMARTER:** We owe it to ourselves, our loved ones, our comrades, our spirituality, our communities, and even our country to be in our best possible physical shape. As men of good character, we can accept that responsibility without question or quibble. A good case study is a group of New York City firefighters who were featured in a series of articles in *USA Today* in the spring of 2000. Twenty-three of the city's bravest went on a weight-reduction program led by Dr. Howard Shapiro, a physician who specializes in weight management. Dr. Shapiro (author of *Dr. Shapiro's Picture Perfect Weight Loss: The Visual Program for Permanent Weight Loss*) showed meal-by-meal trade-offs with roughly the same amount of calories and fat in markedly different compositions. For example, a single 450-calorie fried egg roll was weighed against its caloric equivalent, a full Chinese meal of hot-and-sour soup, scallops, steamed vegetables with a black bean sauce, an orange, and a fortune cookie. These comparisons were made by showing the two food options side by side for visual impact. Several participants in the program lost more than thirty pounds; one guy lost seventy-two pounds. It's a striking and sobering realization that these individuals no doubt bore monumental responsibilities one year later on September 11.

*What this tells us:* Assess your sense of responsibility to family, community, country, God, even your employer and customers. You owe it to all to take good care of yourself.

**2. EDUCATED AND CONFIDENT GUYS MAKE CONSCIOUS FOOD CHOICES:** The incidence of obesity has increased among all age, gender, ethnic, and educational categories in the past ten years. But there is a positive correlation between education and smarter eating habits. This is not surprising to anyone in America, but it's a phenomenon seen in other countries also.

In Finland—an upscale Western country that leads the world in cell phone technologies—nutrition and health awareness are a function of education and the socialization that comes with it. In a study conducted by the National Institute for Consumer Research (Gun Roos, Lysaker, Norway), Finnish engineers and carpenters were questioned on their attitudes about meat and vegetables. The more educated engineers made stronger associations between vegetables and health than did the carpenters; they also seemed to attach pleasure with eating, while the carpenters regarded meals as routine and a provider of fuel. Engineers did not feel that discussing matters of health was a threat to their masculinity, while the carpenters "more actively embrace hegemonic masculinity" (food is a woman's thing). For further insight on hegemony, see item #8 below.

The U.S. Centers for Disease Control found obesity rates that support this finding:

| PERCENT OBESE BY EDUCATION LEVEL | | |
|---|---|---|
| *Group* | *1991* | *2000* |
| Less than high school | 6.5 | 26.1 |
| High school degree | 13.3 | 21.7 |
| Some college | 10.7 | 19.5 |
| College or above | 8.0 | 15.2 |

*What this tells us:* More-educated guys have an advantage; you might lack a degree, but education on nutrition would count the most. However, just because you're a Mr. Smarty Pants doesn't guarantee you're doing it all right.

### 3. GUYS ARE MOTIVATED BY TEAM MEMBERSHIP: For men with a goal, adherence to a well-thought-out eating regimen is more likely. We just have to figure out what we want and devise a plan. From there, it's a matter of following the rules and guidelines we make for ourselves.

Undergraduate male hockey players at the University of Michigan were studied (Smart, Bisogni, Cornell University/University of Michigan), because they were experiencing more food choices in their lives than when they lived at home with their families. As members of a team they had structured schedules, social networks, and performance expectations; they reported that hockey, health, and taste were the factors determining their food practices—health meaning "feeling good for hockey, having a lean and desirable body composition." The study found that such a structure drove better eating habits or "systems," ways of choosing foods that help meet longer-term goals.

*What this tells us:* Join or create a team. It can be a running club, softball team, or basketball league; just get back to your school sport or take up something new. Or start talking about food and nutrition with people at work, perhaps if your employer has a fitness program. If not, get one going or start a smart lunch club. The idea is to find a group of guys who share a performance goal that can be met with healthier eating habits.

**4. GUYS' BODIES ARE PROGRAMMED TO BURN FAT MORE EFFICIENTLY:** Many studies suggest that we are programmed to approach food habits and limitations differently than women—arguably more sensibly, at earlier ages, and not as a function of moods. Why might this be? We're bigger and stronger. We tend to work out differently—we prioritize weight lifting over cardiovascular exercise, although neither should be done exclusively. We have different hormones. We have greater daily food intake needs. We often crave different kinds of food, and some of us, perhaps by nature, respond appropriately to those cravings. It would be a mistake to take any of this to an extreme, but in general it suggests we have advantages women lack.

"In general, we know that men tend to lose weight more easily than women because they have more lean tissue, which is more metabolically active than fat," says Carolyn H. Hollinghsead, Ph.D., R.D., of the College of Health's Division of Foods and Nutrition (University of Utah). And a book published in 2002, *The Testosterone Advantage Plan* (by Lou Schuler, a certified strength and conditioning specialist and fitness director of *Men's Health* magazine), postulates that because men's bodies burn fat differently than women's bodies, we may need to eat more fat. Note that Schuler is speaking to individuals who are fairly serious about fitness and muscular development. It would be a stupid mistake to eat fat to gain muscle if you weren't engaged in a rigorous exercise regimen, and even then it would require very careful measurement and balancing.

In more general terms, the *differences* between men and women—as well as exercisers and sedentary people, young and old people, perhaps even people of different ethnicities and races—are now being considered when it comes to nutrition. "I think we could do a better job of matching up the needs of individuals with the various weight-loss programs available," says Hollingshead, who further suggests that psychological factors probably have a strong role.

*What this tells us:* Exercise to increase lean muscle mass so you can indulge in your natural cravings for fat (just don't take that too far, and learn the differences between smart and dumb fats).

**5. GUYS EAT WITH INTEGRITY:** A study was conducted at Penn State University (Dr. Jennifer Orlet Fish, 1999) that tested how children behave or misbehave when out of parental view with regard to forbidden snack foods. A group of seventy-one kids (three to five years old), thirty-six boys and thirty-five girls, were told that certain foods were off-limits to them, then they were put into an environment where in fact they had free access to the prohibited snacks. An interesting finding: The girls were bad and the boys were good. Says the lead researcher, "For girls only, restricting access predicted girls' snack-food intake, with *higher levels of restriction predicting higher levels of snack-food intake.*" If these characteristics persist to adulthood, this might explain why women on diets seem obsessed with the dessert menus while guys at the same table are checking the Pistons' score.

*What this tells us:* You're not going to kid yourself or anyone else about your eating habits. When you adopt a smarter food structure, it will be an honest venture and one with which you are more likely to stick.

**6. GUYS CAN THINK MULTIDIMENSIONALLY:** We can see beyond the simple metrics of calories and fat grams to consider other essential components of nutrition. We view food and nutrition as part of our whole lives, enabling us to have greater vitality from the inside out. Our motivations aren't always simple . . . well, at least when it comes to weight loss. How can I make such a bold assertion? A study done at the University of Scranton (Oakes, Slotterback 2000) compared men against women on the stereotypes with which each evaluates a food name (not the actual nutrient descriptions). They found that women use less information than men do in selecting a food product. The fairer sex judged food names largely on the basis of fat, while men took vitamins and minerals into account in addition to fat content.

This is particularly encouraging, given the fact that dietary knowledge has evolved in recent years from simplistic good food/bad food generalizations. For example, the difference between processed or simple carbohydrates (table sugar, cake frosting, white rice, pasta) and complex carbohydrates (fruit, vegetables, whole grains, wild rice) is not reflected in simple calorie counts. Men also may be better equipped to make distinctions between certain "good fats" found in nuts, olives, avocados, and cold-water fish (salmon, herring, anchovies, tuna) and "bad fats" found in red meat and processed snack foods.

As packagers of foods strive to meet a federal mandate (by 2006, although many companies will introduce this earlier) to include the amount of "trans fat" (trans-fatty acids derived from hydrogenated vegetable oils) in foods, we should take that factor into account as well— particularly guys who have high cholesterol readings. Just remember that these are packaged foods, processed far from the farm and probably containing copious amounts of simple carbohydrates—a cookie is still a cookie, devoid of antioxidants and fiber. Even a zero trans fat reading doesn't change that.

*What this tells us:* Think before you eat. Employ your native intelligence, what you're learning about nutrition, and what you can derive from food labels and nutrition charts to make your whole life work better. You wouldn't buy a stock, bet on a horse, or argue a political point without due diligence on the facts; you owe yourself the same intellectual respect when it comes to eating smart.

## 7. GUYS DO NOT HAVE TO BE VICTIMS OF CONVENIENCE MARKETING: Sure, the instant gratification of drive-throughs, order-ins, and grab-and-gos will tempt us at every corner, on every commercial break. But we answer to a smarter structure by reaching into our pockets, our refrigerators, or our cupboards for a snack or meal that will sustain us for hours. The potato, grain, and corn syrup industries will do just fine without us. Besides, next time we're playing beach volleyball, will the mega-agribusinesses be there to help us suck in our guts?

*What this tells us:* Be bold and break from the pack. Declare your independence from the convenience culture because *you deserve better.*

## 8. REAL GUYS COOK (AND WOMEN LOVE US FOR IT): The prehistoric discovery of applying heat to food was not necessarily made by a woman. As the physically dominant gender, men almost certainly played a role in building fires and cooking meat. It's time to revisit our roots and refine those skills. The hunting and gathering process is man's work as well—even if it's done online.

According to a study conducted by the University of Minnesota School of Public Health, 27 percent of American men act as primary food handlers for their families. That's right—one-quarter of married guys cook daily for their wife and kids. And not just in the Twin Cities. Husbands in Manhattan interviewed for a story in the *New York Times* seemed to like cooking for their families as much as their wives were eager to relinquish the responsibility. Apparently this is an upward trend, which began in the 1980s.

Lots of men cook. Just look at all the world-famous male chefs: Masculine names populate cookbook titles, food shows, and restaurant rosters. Better yet, many of the newer stars abandon the axiom that a cook has to be a heavyweight to prove his skills.

According to collaborating dietitian Deanna, she and single female friends in Boston place a high premium on men being able to cook. "I would not even entertain the thought of dating a man that did not know how to cook or was unwilling to put a meal together! Many of my friends feel the same way." Our own straw poll of forty women shopping at farmers' markets (see chapter 12) strongly bore this preference out.

*What this tells us:* Cooking can be a guy thing. It draws chicks—and they probably don't even notice how much control it gives you.

**9. TO GUYS, A HOT DOG IS JUST A HOT DOG:** One study of 1,800 obese men and women found that men don't overeat *because of* depression. According to Robert Jeffery, a psychologist at the University of Minnesota, a correlation between depression and overeating exists only in women. This suggests that we just *like* to eat. On the downside, Jeffrey says men tend to be much more overweight than women before they enter a weight-loss program (the study did not determine whether depression or other adverse psychological states *result* when men overeat). This seems to correlate with data that shows that men are disproportionately underrepresented among people with eating disorders such as anorexia and bulimia. Not many guys go into the bathroom after dessert to force themselves to throw up. More likely, we will take our own best advice most of the time, yet allow for Mom's apple pie or a dripping gyro sandwich when a good one comes our way. The trick is not to allow those things to become chronic habits.

*What this tells us:* We should leverage our healthy psychological approach to food by establishing a smart eating structure. When we eat something like deep-fried "elephant ears" on top of a foot-long hot dog at an amusement park, we can joke about it, chase it with a beer—and then regain our dignity with a bowl of oatmeal the next morning.

**10. GUYS' INSTINCTS TO SNACK CAN BE HEALTHY:** Physiological research shows that we are smart to eat snacks in between meals to tide us over; when done right it can keep our energy up and our metabolism cooking along, and reduce gluttony when mealtime comes. The mistake often made is to respond to natural cravings with the wrong foods. Here's how to do it right:

⊃ *Eat Protein Now:* A study from France (Marmonier, et al., Ecole Pratique des Hautes Etudes, 1999) focused on the effects of different types of snacks in forestalling the next meal (the study subjects were young men). Researchers found that a snack highest in protein delayed the desire for dinner by sixty minutes, carbohydrate snacks kept study participants satisfied for only thirty-four minutes, while a chocolate bar (mostly sugar and fat) held them for the least amount of time (twenty-five minutes). A hard-boiled egg or protein bar might be a better choice than, say, buttered popcorn, a Rice Krispie treat, or a chocolate bar.

⊃ *Salt Your Cravings:* At least one study (Leshem, et al., 1998) shows that our taste instincts tell us what we need and we respond appropriately. Male college students at Haifa University, following an hour of exercise, would flavor their soup with 50 percent more salt than before exercising. Researchers speculate "that the immediate and specific increase in NaCl (table salt) preference after exercise is due to sodium loss (in perspiration)." So in this instance, at least, it's natural and metabolically balancing to crave certain things; an erroneous response would be to down an entire bag of barbecue chips or a bag of supersize fries when it's just the salt you need.

*What this tells us:* Cravings are natural. But don't default to the convenience culture (chips, fries, chocolate bars); eat something smarter (beef jerky, broth-based soups, garbanzo beans flavored with Tabasco and lemon juice). Carry smarter snacks with you or know where to find them in stores and fast-food restaurants—these are your best defenses when out on Bad Food Boulevard.

**11. GUYS DON'T HAVE TO ACCEPT FAT AS AN INEVITABLE PART OF AGING:** Weight gain that comes with age is far more a function of reduced physical activity (and therefore less muscle) and deteriorating dietary habits than a law of nature. That fact is illustrated in obesity statistics (U.S. Centers for Disease Control) as segmented by age group:

**PERCENT OBESE BY AGE (U.S., MALE AND FEMALE)**

| Group/age | 1991 | 2000 | Percent change+ |
|-----------|------|------|-----------------|
| 18–29 | 7.1 | 13.5 | 6.4 |
| 30–39 | 11.3 | 20.2 | 8.9 |
| 40–49 | 15.8 | 22.9 | 6.1 |
| 50–59 | 16.1 | 25.6 | 9.5 |
| 60–69 | 14.7 | 22.9 | 8.2 |
| >70 | 11.4 | 15.5 | 4.1 |

The fact that obesity rates are rapidly rising in under-40 age groups shows how factors other than age are at work.

A separate longitudinal study from the U.S. Bureau of Labor Statistics initiated in 1979 found that more than one-quarter of subjects in the study were obese in their late twenties. The people born in 1957 stayed thinner later into life than those born in 1964—Generations X and Y take note.

This situation is part of the reason the American Heart Association released guidelines in July 2002 that recommend assessing risks for heart disease beginning at the age of twenty. "The imperative to prevent the first episode of coronary disease or stroke remains strong because many first-ever heart attacks or strokes are fatal or disabling," says Thomas Pearson, M.D., Ph.D., chairman of the committee that developed this recommendation.

*What this tells us:* Getting older is a flimsy excuse for weight gain; it is a function of bad eating habits and lower activity levels. This should be reason enough to develop a better eating structure at any age.

**12.GUYS KNOW IT'S NOT ANY ONE THING; IT'S EVERYTHING:** We can see how there is no single food that will make us bigger, better, and longer lasting. It's a matter of the whole diet, the whole day, all week and all year. We know that balance, variety, and moderation in our foods bolster all that's good inside us, helping long-term health and vitality in ways that a bowl of orange-colored fish-shaped crackers never could. But if we're stuck in an airport for a few hours late at night, when there is nothing *but* orange fish crackers, it will not kill us to eat a handful (and savor them slowly, one at a time). And we'll track down some real fish, broiled or grilled, the next day.

*What this tells us:* Take a whole-life approach to eating. How you structure your food at home and your approach to eating in routine settings (work lunch or social events) matters far more than what you eat at Thanksgiving dinner or at the annual cannoli festival.

# GOT COKE?

**A**LL THAT FULL-blast sugar soda is stealing stomach room from more nutrient-dense milk. The U.S. Department of Agriculture noted that since the 1970s, teenaged boys have substituted soda for milk in an almost even trade-off: Within this demographic of guys, milk consumption is down by 40 percent and soda is up by the same amount. It's another example of how changing the natural order of life with things like ubiquitous cola machines in schools is a likely explanation for the Guy Paradox. Do these guys pour it on cereal too?

## ATTITUDE CHECK

THE GUY PARADOX MIGHT be the result of other attitudinal factors. Whether or not you would acknowledge such things in yourself, note that these are ideas we've commonly heard from friends.

**Dieting and nutrition is for women.**
Why do women live about seven years longer than men? And during our working years, don't we still compete against those food-perfect women? Maybe a little more information and effort on your part would be a good idea.

**My friends never talk about this stuff.**
You're right, they probably don't. So just be glad you have this book to go to for some sound advice (there's a lot of misinformation out there anyway—you might as well get it from us, a registered dietitian and a guy with a practical approach).

**I'll never be a gourmet cook.**
Again, you are (probably) right. But this is about feeding yourself at

home and making the most of eating out. It's about daily sustenance. You might actually discover how much fun it is to make some decent dishes for a partner and/or friends once you give it a try. But you will not become a gourmet cook from reading this book.

**I'll get better at this when I am older.**

Probably not. Bad habits today will slide into worse habits and sad results a few years later. By then you'll lack energy and motivation. You'll be a slob. You'll be ordering pizza three nights a week and will wonder why you are so bored and tired all the time.

**This is too much to think about.**

No it isn't. If you spend time plotting your next career move or saving for retirement, it is a big miss if you won't be alive for these things. This is your health, longevity, and quality of life we're talking about.

Just as quickly as the Guy Paradox developed, it could disappear. But don't count on government regulation of the food industry or some new miracle pill to do it for you. The responsibility falls squarely on you and your ability to harness your advantages as a guy.

# 7

# a guy's gotta eat foods that taste good

## Leverage your favorite flavors to smarter eating

**The news hardly** gets better than this: Healthy eating and good tastes are inextricably bound—you can't have the former without the latter. But, best of all, you can more or less pig out on some tasty things because they're good for you even in large quantities.

There are many reasons for this, several based in the nature of guys. First, the only way smart food works for guys in the long term is when the food tastes good. We are not oriented to deprivation; we might be able to restrict ourselves to cardboard cuisine for a while, but ultimately we will succumb to nacho cheese, fried chicken, or Ring Dings. We don't automatically calculate calories and fat grams when we look at something; such is the province of the obsessed, which most guys are not. We may have a general sense of the relative healthfulness of, say, fat-free yogurt versus full-fat ice cream, but the real decision usually comes down to what's lip-smackin' good. In other words, the kinds of foods we should learn how to make, or buy when away from home, are those that make us salivate when we think about them.

Second, some of the strong tastes guys tend to like are also the best things for us—flavorings like hot chilies, oregano, citrus juices, vinegar, garlic, onions, olive oil, and even horseradish. Most of these have virtually no fat and no calories, but deliver nutritional benefits, as detailed later in this chapter.

A third bit of happy news: Not all fat is bad. I'm not talking about the reckless, Roman orgy–style decadence of fried onion loaf and shoofly pie. What I mean is that nutritionists now acknowledge that the fat-free goals of the 1990s were too simplistic. The public and the media failed to recognize that there are different kinds of fats with different effects on our health. Instead of just trying to wipe out a macronutrient, fat (and replace it with another macronutrient, carbohydrate), we are now making key distinctions between "good" and "bad" fats. The good fats include those found in peanut butter and most nuts, fattier cold-water fish (salmon, herring, anchovies), olive oil, and avocados (one of the few high-fat vegetables, the primary ingredient of guacamole). Bad fats are the saturated kind found in animal products such as red meats, pork, chicken, and whole-fat milk products. Processed foods made with hydrogenated vegetable oil introduce bad trans-fatty acids to your body. The only plant oils that are saturated are those from the tropics, palm and coconut oil.

From a taste perspective, fat carries flavors. For example, in a grilled salmon the flavors are caramelized with the fat to coat the fish flesh with tastes that can make the mouth water (try lemon with a little salt and pepper). Again, the flavor is in the fats that are actually good for you. In addition, good fats also provide us with nutrients essential to a variety of body functions (including the functions of our brains, of which fat is a major component). But balance, variety, and moderation still need to be adhered to—it's possible to go overboard on any macronutrient, good fats included.

A certain degree of fat is essential to achieving satiety, the state of having had enough. When combined with the other sensory experiences of food such as satisfying flavors, you know you've had a good meal.

# BALANCE, VARIETY, AND MODERATION

**T**HESE WORDS ARE the mantra of dietitians everywhere. It's sort of like hedging your bets—eat a bunch of different things and avoid getting into ruts, and over time things that are not so healthful at least will be mitigated with the good stuff you eat. It sounds reasonable. And part of the beauty of getting variety in your eating is to ease boredom.

A study out of Wageningen University in The Netherlands (Division of Human Nutrition and Epidemiology) found that study subjects who were given the same flavor of meat sauce every night for ten weeks got bored and consumed less over time (groups with varieties of sauces did not reduce consumption as much). That's not terribly surprising. But think of how it can impact the guy who eats the same frozen dinners or simple recipes at home, night after night. He will tend to eat less and then likely gravitate toward something else, such as pizza ordered in or something deplorable from a drive-through.

Develop your skills at cooking a variety of things along with a sense of how to create different flavorings. You'll stick with your structure when it is interesting.

## THERE'S NO ACCOUNTING FOR OTHER PEOPLE'S TASTES

THERE'S CLEAR EVIDENCE THAT taste is personal. What I like, you may hate. And flavors men tend to like are often disdained by women. I learned this at a young age, when my father would get home from his monthly volunteer fire company meetings, an hour or so after my three brothers and I went to sleep. The volunteer firemen, over discussions of barn fires and fund-raisers, had a tradition of eating Limburger cheese with a full slice of onion on rye bread. Nutty, fun guy that my dad was, he would then visit his four sleeping sons to exhale a funky cloud over our pillows. If you're unfamiliar with the smell of Limburger or Limburger breath, think of a running shoe soaked in whole milk and left in a plastic bag on a windowsill for a week in July. I don't remember my mother doing the same thing after fire company women's auxiliary meetings. Whenever she dares to order a spicy menu item in a restaurant, it's the "mild" version. Something called jalapeño poppers caused a bit of a stir a few years ago around our house.

Dads and moms everywhere are simply true to their natures. According to Linda Bartoshuk, Ph.D., a professor at Yale University Medical School who conducts research on the pathologies of taste, a clear difference exists between individuals and genders. People fall into one of three general categories: *supertasters, medium-tasters,* and *non-tasters.* The supertasters constitute about a quarter of the population, and about two-thirds of that quarter are women. From this we can generalize that women are more likely to be supertasters, while us guys skew toward the medium- or non-taster categories.

Supertasters are particularly sensitive to tastes, as the name suggests. They will find some tastes too strong, while blander foods are satisfying to them. Because we guys lack this taste sensitivity, we tend to find blandness unsatisfying.

The business of taste relative to gender gets interesting when you consider the pain/pleasure dynamic of "picante," or hot, spicy foods. Dr. Bartoshuk's research found fewer clear gender distinctions on the preference for pain/pleasure (relative to gastronomy). But she did note that men who have duller taste sensors (medium- to non-tasters), require more spicy ingredients to stimulate our pain/pleasure. In other words, most guys who like it hot will require a greater quantity of hot sauce than most women to get the same response.

Food choices and flavoring preferences are both personal and often different from that of the opposite sex, for physiological reasons. That Tabasco television commercial from a few years ago, with the backwoods guy sitting on a porch, eating pizza doused in hot sauce that ultimately caused blood-sucking mosquitoes to explode, was to me like looking in a mirror. I love hot sauce on pizza. Lots of it. But maybe you don't. How do you know what your own personal taste preferences might be? It's simple—think of your favorite foods. If you like pizza, it might be because of the tanginess of the sauce, or perhaps because of the texture and taste of the cheese. Maybe you like sweet-and-sour soup, which also has a certain tang. For me, Buffalo chicken wings taste great in part because the fatty skin on the chicken, the hot sauce, and the blue-cheese dressing on the side make a great (fatty) combination (I indulge in wings two or three times a year).

# TEXTURE: MORE THAN A FEELING

**Y**OUR MOUTH TELLS you two things about the food you're eating: what it tastes like, and how it feels. The sensory experience of eating involves the texture as well as the taste of food. Babies, incapacitated hospital patients, and a few other categories of people eat only mushy foods. The rest of us enjoy a mix of textures, which *The Elements of Taste* (Kunz, Kaminsky) likens to punctuation: "Crunch is a signal to stop one taste experience and start another, kind of like a period in a sentence. Smoothness, which rounds out tastes, works like a comma, extending the experience of tasting." Michael Carmel, director of Culinary Arts at the Illinois Institute of Art Culinary Arts School, explains it in the context of the whole menu item. "You want to layer flavors and textures for a full sensory experience." To me, a multitextured dish elicits what dietitians tell us we should get in our diets: balance, variety, and moderation. A BLT sandwich might have unhealthy bacon, but my mouth also feels whole-grain bread, lettuce, and tomato, which as a whole seems like a smart meal. Even a party buffet might allow us to eat greasy chips with fatty dips (a much better choice would be salsa), but by also including celery and carrot sticks, the evening isn't a complete dietary disaster.

Also, I seem to be drawn to acidic tastes (citrus juices, vinegar), maybe because I was raised with German cooking (sauerbraten, German-style potato salad, vinegar-based coleslaw, sauerkraut). Most people develop taste preferences from what they were fed early in life. If you have a passion for drive-through fast food, you probably have been conditioned to like a lot of salt and grease, plus the carbs in French fries and hamburger buns. Or maybe, like me, you discovered that a basic hamburger tasted best with lots of ketchup, mustard, and a pickle—in other words, the toppings were a big part of what did it for you.

Certain foods are known to be preferred more by men than by women. According to consumption patterns studied by the U.S. Department of Agriculture:

⊃ Guys consume 58.7 percent of all tomato products (whole, sauce, juice, and ketchup), even though we make up slightly less than 49 percent of the population.

⊃ Men eat 53 percent of (fresh) bell peppers, and those in the 20–39 age group eat 24 percent of peppers even though they constitute only 16 percent of the population.

⊃ Male consumers have a stronger preference for fresh apples than women, who prefer applesauce and dried apples.

⊃ Men consume about 40 percent more onions than women.

Each of these foods stands on its own, but all are used to add flavor to larger recipes—three of the four often turn up on a pizza.

When you come to discover the flavors you like the most, you're on your way to learning how to enjoy new and healthier foods. A study out of the University of Toronto (Pliner, Stallberg-White, 1998) found that children are more willing to try new foods (a different type or flavor of chip) when served in combination with a familiar taste (a chip dip they already knew and liked). This implies that the familiar helps usher in the unfamiliar. So if you like the sour taste of lemon juice and the bite of black pepper, for example, but are not sure about grilled salmon, put all three together and your chances for acquiring a preference for this very healthful fish are increased.

Here are a few other approaches to taste transfer:

⊃ Mix a little melted butter with hot sauce and drizzle it over a mash of tuna and corn, topped with Parmesan cheese. It has the mouthwatering taste of Buffalo chicken wings, but delivers protein with less fat.

⊃ Do you have an addiction to a specific flavor of potato chips? Substitute edamame (soybeans in the pod) for chips and you get a protein-filled snack with healthy, plant-based fats instead.

Edamame comes frozen by the bag; fill a small bowl with some, then mix in the flavors you find addictive and microwave for a minute or two. Try a little vinegar, olive oil, and salt (salt and vinegar); barbecue spices (barbecue); or hot sauce (jalapeño). You don't eat the pod, but squeeze it through your front teeth to pop out the soybeans, tasting the flavor from the husks.

If you don't like the bitterness of tea, a squeeze of lime or other fruit juice makes it much more drinkable. Green tea is strongly associated with lower incidences of certain cancers, especially those of the esophagus (for which people with acid reflux disease are at risk).

## TASTES TO LOVE

IN CHAPTER 10, WE will break down the components of smart cooking into three parts: *Main Stuff, Flavor,* and *Crunch.* Main Stuff and Crunch often (but not always) lack a distinct taste. Rarely does one eat chicken, fish, broccoli, or green beans without something to flavor them. Applied heat will bring out some flavors—a process called caramelizing, turning a food's inherent sugars and amino acids to carbon, seen in the grill marks on barbecued meat and grilled vegetables or the dark parts of burnt toast. But added flavors like salt, pepper, or garlic are what your senses notice first and most. Your goal then is to apply an interesting flavor (e.g., salt, lemon juice, oregano, steak sauce, berries) to taste-bland Main Stuff or Crunch (e.g., tuna, cauliflower, cottage cheese, beans), such that you can enjoy healthier foods and consequently eat them regularly. You might follow the recipes provided later in this book to the letter. But you'll live long and prosper, as a guy, when you experiment beyond this book. After all, taste is personal (not everyone loves steak sauce on cottage cheese and beans, much to my puzzlement).

The food scientists who devise spicy fries, special sauces, and specialty potato chips know all this. It's that old free-enterprise thing at work again—they find ways of making cheap commodity goods such as potatoes taste great with salt, fat, and natural and artificial flavors. Peruse the ingredient labels on non-diet beverages at the grocery store—they are mostly just variations on water and high-fructose corn syrup. In your own kitchen, you will probably do better because you can create tastes that only you will love.

Taste can come from good-for-you as well as less-good-for-you things. On the downside are butter, fats, sugar, and excessive salt. Ask anyone who cooks a Thanksgiving meal—just about every dish on the table calls for a stick or two of butter (except the cranberries and Jell-O). But sometimes butter is the only taste that will do; on toast, for example. So understand that all tastes are fine in moderation; your bigger concern is the main meal—if you have to butter your green beans to like them, then go ahead and do that. The beautiful thing is how many great tastes are low in (or free of) calories or fat. Many even carry nutritional benefits.

The following list, Guys' Great Tastes, provides ideas and reasons to start taking personal control of your food. Note the variety, and that most of these foods have long shelf lives (some last for years in my kitchen because a small quantity will do).

## GUYS' GREAT TASTES

MOST OF THESE FLAVORING agents are like a little dose of health added to a meal; in some cases, adding them is like taking vitamins with breakfast. Here's a quick review of the functional and nutritional characteristics of these flavors:

**CITRIC JUICE:** Citric juices add zing to just about anything—I even squeeze a lime over my turkey chili. My simplest all-protein snack is a frozen chicken breast in a bowl with about a half-inch of lemon juice, sprinkled with black pepper and oregano; microwave for about seven minutes (more or less depending on your oven strength; flip the chicken after four minutes), then eat. Now scrape the brown stuff from the sides of the bowl and taste it. Yummy. Citrus is also good as a salt substitute, which is important to individuals needing to reduce sodium (for example, people suffering from hypertension and other heart conditions, or kidney conditions). Bottled citric juices are relatively interchangeable and have a long shelf life. Lemon and lime are also high in vitamin C—which has the well-known benefits of preventing scurvy, helping the immune response to colds and other germs, and strengthening collagen.

**VINEGAR:** Another acidic zinger, vinegar tastes so good to me that I often drink a capful or two while cooking. It's a strong flavor, however, and it's easy to use too much. Vinegar comes in dozens of varieties; red wine, apple cider, or malt versions carry plenty of taste, but the rich, dark balsamic is truly guy gourmet. Hippocrates advocated vinegar as a medicine, a use the holistic crowd espouses even today (most purported medical benefits have not been adequately studied).

**TABASCO AND CRUSHED CHILI PEPPERS:** Made largely from hot peppers, vinegar, salt, and sometimes tomatoes, onions, and garlic, hot sauces are definitively strong tastes that work for simple cooks like myself. It's best to hold off adding these sauces until you're ready to eat, just to make sure you don't overdo it. With practice, you can learn how adding crushed chili peppers to a stew or other recipe can permeate the entire dish, leaving a pleasant aftertaste that lingers and improves your satiety. Some small studies suggest that the active component of chili peppers, capsaicin, raises metabolism during and after a meal to the extent that it actually helps you burn extra calories. It should also be noted that capsaicin derived from pepper is now also marketed as a topical pain reliever.

**OREGANO:** An herb I first encountered in a wax packet accompanying a pizza delivery, this is a spice favored by Italians, Greeks, and people of other cultures throughout the Mediterranean. Its name derives from the Greek for "joy of the mountains." Perhaps it works well for guys in a broad variety of foods (egg dishes, anything involving beans, chicken) because we're reliving happy memories of pizzas past. Among herbs, it has one of the highest concentrations of antioxidants. Historically, it has been touted (but not necessarily proven through research) to ameliorate everything from digestive disturbances, constipation, diarrhea, parasitic infections, coughs, headaches, menstrual irregularities, and bacterial and viral infections. (But if you have menstrual irregularities, you *seriously* need to see a doctor.)

**SALT AND PEPPER:** Few tastes are as basic and universal as salt and its table-top cousin, pepper. According to *The Elements of Taste*, "Salt is the king of tastes," which the author speculates has something to do with our evolutionary roots. We usually get too much salt in processed foods and that's of particular concern to people who have hypertension or high blood pressure (two of my brothers were diagnosed in their thirties). Regardless, salt enhances all other flavors, while peppers of all kinds (black, chili, cayenne, pimento, paprika) trigger a pain/pleasure response on the tongue (a good thing).

**SWEETENERS (SUGAR, HONEY, ASPARTAME, ETC.):** When in the American South, if you ask for unsweetened iced tea what you get is a dirty look. Some people just have to have it sweet. Sugar of course adds calories (the same goes for honey), but that's not such a horrible thing if it gets you to enjoy fruit more. It's far better for you to take in sixteen calories from a packet of sugar sprinkled on a grapefruit than to never eat grapefruit. Sugar isn't just for sweet foods, either—check the label of many non-sweet products such as ketchup or tomato sauce and you'll see some form of sugar pretty high up on the list. For more on the choices you have in sweetening, see page 49.

**PARMESAN AND ROMANO CHEESES (GRATED):** Cheeses of all types, including these two, are made mostly of fat, sodium, and protein. In excess, that can work against you because of the artery-clogging effects of saturated fat. But the beauty of these cheeses, sprinkled lightly on foods, is that a little bit goes a long way. They're a no-brainer on tomato-based foods, but also go well on steamed vegetables, egg dishes, and green salads. The flavor, mixed with lemon juice on something like cauliflower, asparagus, or broccoli, is food for the gods.

**PREPARED SALAD DRESSING (LOWER-FAT VERSIONS):** You can pretty much ignore everything else you read in this chapter and go the easy route by putting manufactured salad dressings on a lot of foods. They're not just for green salads, you know. Do you see all those floaty things at the bottom of the bottle? Those are herbs, spices, and onion bits—all tastes that mix well together. Also, commercial salad dressings have ingredients like xanthan gum, calcium disodium edta, and hydro-genated vegetable oil, the amount of which might be reduced as awareness of trans-fatty acids grows. Certain varieties also have lots of sugar (this bothers me a little). But the easiest healthy meal you can make at the end of a long day is nuked meat, steamed vegetables, and low-fat oil-based dressing over everything. The only trouble is that I like to come up with my own tastes, because prepared salad dressings can get boring after a while. So when making a meal for other people, try mixing a dose or two of olive oil with an equal amount of vinegar and a few spices (rosemary, pepper, salt, oregano, cilantro, or whatever) for a fresh salad dressing.

**OLIVE OIL:** It's almost all fat (made up of a mixture of polyunsaturated and monounsaturated fats—which are the good fats and which explains why olive oil gets so much press), and it doesn't taste like much on its own. Yet olive oil is perhaps the most important ingredient for anything you cook in a skillet. Oil (in addition to olive, also try flaxseed, peanut, corn, or canola) is a medium for other tastes to emerge, providing a means for spices, meats, and vegetables to cook and caramelize without burning. Oil also helps absorption of other nutrients, like vitamin E. Vegetable oils are like meat lard in that they are mostly fat, but unlike animal fats, which are saturated, most vegetable oils are composed of mono- or polyunsaturated fat—the good fat. Note that for simple frying, the spray versions of olive oil and butter help reduce total consumption.

**ONIONS:** Talk about packing a punch in small amounts. The most common onions are red (which are best used uncooked in salads, sandwiches, and on burgers) and yellow (which deliver more taste when stir-fried). Onions have a strong taste that works in a variety of raw and cooked meals. Like other fruits and vegetables, onions contain specific components (quercetin and the antioxidant selenium) that have known health-promoting benefits. From a study published in November 2002 in the *Journal of the National Cancer Institute* (Hsing, et al.), high marks go to scallions, garlic, onions, leeks, chives, and shallots (all related vegetables) for their strong association with the prevention of prostate cancer, one of the most common forms of cancer in men. The flavonols present in this group collectively known as allium are also linked to lower incidences of cancers of the stomach, colon, and esophagus.

**MINCED GARLIC:** Like the name says, it's garlic prechopped for you. Now, you could save money if you bought whole garlic by itself and did all the chopping. But your hands would stink for days. *Garlic is a good food.* Like many herbal and plant foods, there is broad folklore espousing benefits of garlic that have yet to be verified by scientific study. It might work as an antifungal, moderate blood pressure, reduce "bad" cholesterol, improve circulation, mitigate impotence, work as a "cardioprotective" and an antioxidant, relieve coughs and colds, and help stomach conditions. As with most traditional folk remedies and preventives, the economics required to conduct extensive, long-term research on the benefits of garlic is lacking. Some university research—interestingly, much more of it conducted in Europe and Canada than in the United States—validates garlic's ability to fight high cholesterol and heart disease, as well as the antibacterial properties of allicin, an active component of garlic. A distant relative of mine who lived well into her nineties claimed her longevity was due to her eating a clove of garlic every day. You just didn't want to spend too much time with her in close quarters. Regarding the breath thing, there are ways to combat it—parsley or breath mints after dinner—but the stuff lingers in your bloodstream and stomach gases, which strikes me as a further indication of a pervasive health effect. As a rule, don't eat or serve it on a date unless both parties agree to do it together (a "stink pact").

**CILANTRO:** This is a love it or hate it taste. Personally, I can't get enough of the stuff—it goes great with anything involving tomatoes or avocados (such as in guacamole), mixed with green salads, and chopped over grilled meat. As a green, leafy ingredient, it should be added late in the cooking process—if not after the main meal is removed from heat, just before serving. It has a unique, if not overpowering, flavor. Lots of Web sites promote it as a digestive aid and to prevent infections, which seem to be the purported benefits of anything herbal (ginger, garlic, etc.).

**MUSTARDS:** I grew up in the era of basic hot dog mustard, but now, for better or worse, we have choices ranging from the swank Grey Poupon to my favorite earthy, grainy German-style mustards. Its spiciness is best kept in check, so don't overdo it; but it is possible to eat mustard on most meats (including fish), vegetables, and eggs. Mix it in with olive oil and vinegar for extra kick in a salad dressing. It says something about a taste when it has a history of use in clearing the sinuses and increasing blood flow (mustard plasters). Although never used in quantities large enough to matter, mustard is typically free of fat and cholesterol. Just don't be fooled by "Dijonnaise" or other forms of mustard that are largely mayonnaise; this labeling trick fooled a lot of people when it was first introduced in the fat-phobic 1990s.

**HORSERADISH:** Served at Passover seders to represent the suffering of the Jews under Pharaoh's rule, horseradish is to northern Europeans what chilies are to Latin Americans and people of certain Asian cultures— at its best when you feel a rush up the back-side of the head. I was fed horseradish in my formative years on roast-beef-and-weck sandwiches (the culinary brainchild of Buffalo that preceded hot chicken wings); now I put it on anything that I like, including bland submarine sandwiches I buy at a convenience store near where I live. I do this intuitively, but some evidence indicates that the allyl isothiocyanate present in both horseradish and mustards might fight bacteria such as *E. coli* in meats.

**STEAK SAUCE:** This is in the category of "commercial products you could make yourself, but why bother?"—much like prepared salad dressings and seasoning packets. It elicits a strong association with something you already know and presumably like—grilled steak—which you then can transfer over to something new (fish, chicken, or a vegetable). Manufacturers of steak sauce sporadically promote it for non-steak use. Perhaps tuna or brussels sprouts with steak sauce might not trip your wire, but try it to see if you like it. The various commercial brands vary in taste, of course; most are made with tomato purée, vinegar, salt, and sugars, each of which is relatively benign in small quantities.

**PREPARED SPICE BLENDS (IN DRY PACKS):** Again, someone with the time and inclination could throw together a lot of spices on his own, but sometimes convenience can't be beat. Prepared spice blends can be added to any dish that would otherwise take salt (for example, a bean dish), or used for its intended purposes, stated on the product label. There are dozens of different varieties of dry pack mixes—find the ones that appeal to you most. Here's a real *A Guy's Gotta Eat*-style recipe from Mrs. Dash, a brand I sometimes buy:

*Carrot Salad:* One pound carrots, grated; one tablespoon Mrs. Dash Onion & Herb Seasoning; ½ cup raisins; ½ cup walnuts, chopped; one cup yogurt with fruit, low-fat; one tablespoon brown sugar. Toss grated carrots, raisins, walnuts. Mix together yogurt, Mrs. Dash Onion & Herb Seasoning, and brown sugar; add to carrot mixture and mix well; cover and refrigerate. Preparation time: approximately five minutes. Cooking time: none.

Note that neither I, nor anyone I know, works for Mrs. Dash. I simply respect a recipe that is healthy, easy, quick, and tastes good (it gets extra points for an unusual mix of ingredients). This recipe is also a good demonstration of how a mix of sugar, salt, and spice makes for an appealingly complex taste.

**CINNAMON:** I put it on grapefruit and in anything involving apples. More broadly, people of many cultures add it to any fruit, including the odd-but-healthy category of "fruit soups" (different fruits mixed, sometimes with milk), as well as the rice puddings favored by German and Scandinavian cooks. Cinnamon is purported to prevent tooth decay and ease stomach irritation.

**BERRIES:** Most fruit adds flavor to a dish; little chopped-up bits of apple on a green salad would wow any dinner guest because it's a cheap and easy way to add taste complexity. But berries can be your best buddies for a number of reasons. First, raspberries, blueberries, strawberries, and their exotic cousins (mulberries, blackberries, bilberries, and elderberries) have distinct flavors that can make morning oatmeal, a protein shake, or a yogurt dessert pretty darn interesting. Second, frozen varieties are just as tasty and easy to get all year. Researchers are now finding that blueberries in particular, and perhaps other berries as well, help slow the aging process of the neurological system. So berries at breakfast might help you to remember how to eat smart the rest of the day *and* keep your hook shot on the basketball court.

# COLOR MY BRAIN

**N**UTRITIONISTS NOW SAY that what we *see* is linked to better nutrition as well. Multiple studies tie components that help eyesight (vitamin A, carotenoids, anthocyanins and other flavonoids, betalains, and chlorophyll—all good stuff, much of which is linked to cancer prevention) directly to plant pigments.

Early in the twentieth century, richly colored vegetables (yellow corn, carrots, and sweet potatoes) were found to reduce symptoms of vitamin A deficiencies, while bland-colored produce (white corn and parsnips) did not. A notable exception is dark red beets, which score low on vitamin A, but are still a good source of folate, potassium, and fiber. (I hated beets as a kid and called them "poison fish"; my enthusiasm for them today remains muted).

*The Color Code* (coauthored by James A. Joseph, Ph.D., Chief of the Neuroscience Laboratory at the USDA Human Nutrition Research Center on Aging at Tufts University, and Daniel Nadeau, M.D., in March 2002) extols findings on blueberries. "My experience in the area of aging research and more specifically my most recent work with blueberries has made me a believer in pigment power," says Dr. Joseph. "We've always known that fruits and vegetables are good for you, but now we're starting to find out why. The natural compounds that make blueberries blue or spinach green are powerful allies in the fight against aging." This further reinforces the importance of fruits and vegetables, which are some of the most brightly colored products of nature. What the caveman ate while walking through the woods—carrots, apples, watermelon, peas, blueberries—were the things that visually jumped out at him. It's nature's way of keeping us in the pink.

**SPICY GARDEN MIX:** Got a sandwich, vegetable, or other boring dish? Give it some kick and crunch with pickled and peppery vegetables. This basically combines two of my favorite tastes, vinegar and chilies, with small chunks of cauliflower, cucumbers, carrots, celery, and onions. A popular submarine sandwich chain offers this as one of their toppings, for which I frequently ask.

**GINGER ROOT:** You are not going to believe how talented you are when you figure out how to slice some fresh ginger into your food. Ginger has a sharp bite; perhaps you've tasted it as the pink stuff served alongside the green stuff in a sushi restaurant. Added to chicken in the last few minutes of cooking, it delivers a surprising little charge—ginger almost qualifies as a pepper. Like many other herbs and roots, it supposedly relieves indigestion. Note that the fresh form is a brown, hairy, gnarled tuber thing, with a surprisingly long shelf life (available in the produce section—it also comes in powdered and packaged form). Ginger is one of those ingredients used in Asian cultures to fix just about every health condition (too numerous to list here).

**SUN-DRIED TOMATOES:** Someone somewhere goes to a lot of trouble slicing and drying tomato halves, but it's pretty amazing what happens when he or she does. Like any dried fruit or vegetable, a big quantity of the tomato shrinks (mostly by moisture loss) so that the remaining taste is concentrated, rich, and intense. And we guys like intense flavors. Since most sun-dried tomatoes are used in foods requiring a little oil (salads, chicken dishes), I suggest you buy the "in oil" variety versus the dried packages (you have to add oil to those anyway to get them to work in dishes). As detailed earlier, tomatoes are a good source of lycopene, a component that acts as an antioxidant and is associated with the prevention of prostate cancer.

**BASIL:** This is a leafy green that has a distinctive flavor you might have tasted in combination with sliced tomatoes and goat cheese. A guy cooking for himself is unlikely to use basil on an everyday basis; I certainly don't. But for guests, if you want a cheap and easy wow for your meal, get a bag or bunch of basil in the fresh produce section of the grocery store. Chop it up and sprinkle it on cooked meats or vegetables, or add it to a green salad. According to MotherNature.com, "In Japan, India, and West Africa, various species of basil are used to treat colds, flu, fevers, joint pain, stomach cramps, nausea, and headaches."

**SALSA:** A surprising food fact from a few years ago was how salsa sales surpassed those of ketchup. Beyond its simple tomato base, salsa has all kinds of other vegetable ingredients (tomatillos, onions, chilies, cilantro, and garlic, to name a few) that add crunch and flavor and quite a few vitamins as well (usually with no fat). Salsa is a quick way to turn anything zesty, and it's far more versatile than ketchup and chip dip, the junk food it replaces. You might even declare a Salsa Week: Try it on everything from cabbage to eggs, chicken, and fish, just to see what it can do.

There's no need to stop with these great tastes. Start paying attention to what other people serve at home or in independently owned restaurants (the chains rarely venture from the tried-and-true because they tend to market to the least venturesome diners). You owe it to yourself and the quality of your life to find the food flavors you enjoy the most.

## INTERACTIVITY AND COMPLEXITY

WE GUYS LIKE TO present ourselves as simple. We like our beer, our TV, and some good grub. It's all a lie. We are highly evolved organisms, and what we eat betrays this not-so-simple truth. Take our sandwiches, for instance. A basic peanut butter and jelly or grilled cheese might be quick, easy, and not so bad in the health department (much better than a frozen pizza popover, anyway). But life is a little more grand with a Dagwood-style late-night sandwich, piled three or more inches high with bread, meat, cheese, greens, and condiments ranging from mustard to mayo to horseradish.

We like our food layered and crunchy, multiflavored and hearty. And we like to feel full when we are done. This is because we intuitively understand the ways different foods interact with each other; the complexity of different tastes provides our palates with a complete sensory experience—and nutrition. Broken down into individual components, sandwiches are full, healthy meals of whole-grain carbohydrates (bread), protein (meat, chicken, fish, or peanut butter), vegetables (lettuce, tomatoes, pickles, pickled peppers) and maybe even fruit (jam, which goes with much more than just peanut butter). The same can be said for our other favorites: one-skillet wonders, supreme pizzas, and burritos.

# FOOD THROUGH THE NOSE AND EYES

**D**O YOU THINK taste is all about the mouth? You're wrong. The nose is as important to the enjoyment of food as the tongue. The pleasure of food begins even before the aroma reaches us. "We taste first with our eyes, then the nose, then the tongue," says Renée Zonka, professor of nutritional cooking in the culinary school of the Illinois Institute of Art. Like most accomplished chefs, Renée teaches students how to "plate" the food in a way that is attractive, an essential part of the sensory experience.

From that standpoint, we're really gourmets deep down inside. Pick up a cookbook, turn on the Food Network, or talk to any chef and you will discover the symphony of sensory input in a good dish. Guys mix foods together just because we like it.

The person who first woke me up to this was Susan Stamberg, correspondent on National Public Radio's "All Things Considered." Every Thanksgiving, she offers the listening audience her mother-in-law's cranberry relish recipe, which includes coarsely ground cranberries, an onion, sour cream, sugar, and horseradish. I remember her saying, "This is where it gets weird" before explaining the horseradish part. I am recipe-averse, but the words "weird" and "horseradish" together piqued my interest. I had previously worried that my strange experiments with cans and bottles and bags of things from the far corners of the kitchen were the concoctions of a demented cheap-ass. But that radio broadcast was the moment I realized that mine was a visionary fusion of fruits from a bountiful land—albeit canned fruits past their expiration date. (The cranberry relish recipe is available on the NPR.org Web site.)

In summary, what this means for the subsistence-level cook is that you should feel free to experiment, to put unusual stuff together. If you like anchovies and you think they'll go well in, say, a fruit salad, have at it. If you, like me, want to mix peanut butter with just about everything, go forth and spread it. Heck, if the Thais can put peanut butter on chicken and the Dutch can melt it with mayonnaise onto fried potatoes, why can't I drizzle it on orange slices?

Be the food. Make it you. It's all about pushing the envelope.

# EATING OUT:
# DON'T BE CONFINED BY CONDIMENTS

**Y**OU CAN'T ALWAYS have it your way. Whether at fast-food or fancy white-tablecloth restaurants, much of the flavoring is determined long before you pull into the parking lot. That's because the restaurants get most of their foods par-baked and pre-spiced from suppliers, the economics of food service requiring that such activities take place at a manufacturing site instead of labor-expensive retail settings. But you can use some discretion in your choice of condiments. Rules of thumb:

■ Mayonnaise comes in many flavors: "Horsey sauce" and even "horseradish" in several fast-food chains are largely mayonnaise, with all the fat that comes with it. Chicken sandwiches lose their low-fat advantage over beef burgers once the creamy white mayo hits the bun. "Special sauce" is basically mayonnaise with other things tossed in, and the virtuous submarine sandwich suffers the same fate if you choose one of the creamy sauces they offer (choose vinaigrette or just vinegar).

■ Ketchup, mustard, and relish beat out mayo, but beware the "dijonnaise" mayos, which were a ploy of the food industry in recent years to wed the perception of low-fat mustard with high-fat mayo.

■ Look for and eschew restaurant menu items that say "creamy." Creamy is usually one form or another of dairy fat.

■ Asian restaurants' sauces (soy, plum, hot mustard) are usually quite healthy, except for the high salt content (to be avoided by people with high blood pressure).

Still not satisfied? Here's a trick I use at my favorite burrito bar: I swipe a few lemons from the beverage area (intended for iced-tea drinkers) and squeeze them onto my fajita along with a jigger or two of hot sauce. The very tangy taste is supremely satisfying.

# PART II

# GET EQUIPPED

**SOMETHING** about our culture places a higher value on things you can enjoy at home. We watch rented movies on big-screen TVs in our living rooms instead of going to the cineplex. At-home gyms are bought by phone. Bathrooms are built with steam jets and Jacuzzis to replicate spas. And the Internet lets you buy cars, groceries, music, and books in your underwear. So why shouldn't food—pretty high on the physical needs list—be there and ready to cook in your home as well?

Actually, there are more men cooking today than ever before. Blame women's liberation. Or maybe men's liberation? Guys who cook might think of it as a control thing. It doesn't matter—being able to make your own dinner is as much about convenience as it is about making meals that taste great and keep you fit.

Your first move is to get the right tools, then the provisions. Because like a boy scout, a guy's gotta be prepared.

# 8

# a guy's gotta prep his kitchen

## The essential tools of the cave

**Half of your meals,** on average, will or should be eaten at home. How can you do that if you don't have the proper equipment and supplies? Stocking up with the right stuff will considerably advance your health and well-being. Because you are battling a culture that wants you to choose a false sense of convenience over your own health and appearance, think of this in combative terms. You are waging a war of independence from bad convenience food. Your weapon is a well-armed kitchen.

To get started, here's what you'll need:

**Resolve.** You have to *believe*, man. You *can* eat smart (and improve your social functionality as a party-giver) with equipment, supplies, and know-how.

**About $300 (add another $300 for the food).** In case this seems like a lot to you, keep in mind that these are durable goods that can last a decade or longer. Amortized, that would be about $30 per year toward being healthier. Alternatively, if you eat every meal out (breakfast for $7, lunch for $8, and dinner for around $10, for a daily total of $25), you are spending about $750 per month. And you have no blender or skillet at the end of the day to show for it.

You could get away with spending much less. Instead of buying kitchen utensils, you could (a) get them from generous/concerned family and friends as gifts; (b) assiduously search the sales, in Sunday newspaper advertisements or online; or (c) go to yard sales, second-hand stores, dollar stores, warehouse/club stores, and flea markets, where you could pay 5 percent of the regular price. Another ploy is to play off the sympathy and delirium of friends who are about to get married. They will be getting all new stuff through their own scam, shower and wedding gifts, so snare their old utensils as the new ones arrive.

**Two hours.** It will take more time if you like to comparison-shop between stores, less if you do it online. Note that you can combine your shopping trip for utensils with your first grocery trip. Just get the utensils first. A kettle will fare better for a few hours in the trunk than yogurt and frozen chicken breasts.

## THE BIG TWELVE OF THE CAVEMAN KITCHEN

IT'S A SMART IDEA to get it all in one fell swoop. The caveman forged his tools from bones, sticks, rocks, and God knows what else; fortunately, modern technology and merchandising bring us our utensils with relative ease and affordability, free of vertebrate remains.

The following items are essentially what I've found to be most versatile and effective. I have some pretty ugly, well-worn utensils from this list that continue to work fine after years of use. A selection of optional items is included, but none is absolutely necessary.

This list assumes you have basic serving implements (plates, bowls, cutlery/flatware, drinking glasses) and standard kitchen appliances (refrigerator/freezer, stove, and microwave; the oven itself is a place for storing nonflammable items). If you do not have a microwave, go out and buy one. Many are priced at less than $100; this component is essential.

## 1. CAN OPENER

*Primary Function:* Opening cans, something you will do a lot.

*Look for:* Hand-driven models are best; electric versions work fine, but take up space, are harder to clean, and are more expensive.

*Maintenance:* Rinse after each use; run through the dishwasher occasionally.

*Commonly Priced at:* Under $12.

## 2. DEEP SKILLET (A.K.A. FRYING PAN, CHEF'S PAN)

*Primary Function:* Cooking meats, vegetables, and soups. Also available in smaller sizes, often sold economically as a set, but a large one is all you need for subsistence cooking.

*Look for:* Most types have nonstick coatings (Teflon, T-fal, and others), a feature you will appreciate. However, even with careful use many frying surfaces will wear off; if that bothers you, pricier pans with ultra-smooth metal surfaces (Scan Pan, All-Clad) reportedly work as well and last longer. A glass lid makes it easier to check in on things; however, you probably will need to stir the food to avoid burning, which of course requires lifting the lid anyway.

*Maintenance:* For nonstick pans, be sure to use nonmetal spatulas and spoons. Dishwasher-appropriate, although its size might make it easier to hand-wash with nonabrasive scrubbing pads (see manufacturer's instructions).

*Commonly Priced at:* Under $50; entire sets of skillets, saucepans, and other kettles and pots are sold starting at under $100.

## 3. SAUCEPAN

*Primary Function:* Cooking juicy/soupy things, like soups, chili's and stews, rice, pasta, hot bean dishes, and hard-boiled eggs. Also serves as companion to the steamer insert (see next item).

*Look for:* It should be at least four inches deep and seven inches in diameter; bigger is OK. Should come with a lid.

*Maintenance:* Wash after each use; run through the dishwasher occasionally.

*Commonly Priced at:* Under $30 (see deep skillet pricing above regarding sets).

## 4. STEAMER INSERT

*Primary Function:* Steaming vegetables.

*Look for:* This is the thing with holes in it that sits over boiling water, often set in a saucepan. Very cheap versions can last a long time (I purchased one for about $5 in the early 1980s and it has lasted a full twenty years). Some saucepans are sold with these; best if stainless steel.

*Maintenance:* Dishwasher-safe.

*Commonly Priced at:* Around $15 and up.

## 5. LARGE KETTLE (A.K.A. STOCK POT, CASSEROLE)

*Primary Function:* To cook soups, stews, larger-quantity pastas, and rice (for entertaining) and just as a second saucepan when you have several things to make. Also serves as a fine bucket for icing bottled beverages consumed away from the kitchen (on a patio or deck, for example).

*Look for:* About ten inches high and nine inches in diameter, or bigger.

*Maintenance:* Wash after each use; it's probably too big for the dishwasher.

*Commonly Priced at:* Around $40 and up, also available within sets (see deep skillet).

## 6. ONE GREAT KNIFE

*Primary Function:* Slicing things (fresh fruit and vegetables, meat and cheese).

*Look for:* Straight-edge blade (nonserrated; the toothy kind is more for use on breads, cakes, and muffins, all things not to have around the house anyway), approximately ten inches (handle base to blade tip). Handle should be sturdy and resilient (when a knife breaks, it's almost always the handle).

*Maintenance:* Wash with hot, soapy water in between cutting different types of food (especially meat); dishwasher-safe (non-wood handles).

*Commonly Priced at:* A single, quality knife can range $20–75. This is a workhorse item, so spending a little extra can be worth it. Optional and advised is a knife sharpener (manual, costing about $20). Another option is the chef's set of multiple items (costing as little as $40); the drawback is that they might be of lower quality and include several items you probably will not need (deboner, paring knife, bread knife).

## 7. CUTTING BOARD (POLYETHYLENE, STONE, OR GLASS ONLY)

*Primary Function:* Slicing things, including vegetables, fruit, and meat.

*Look for:* The hard-surface board (versus wood, which is porous) is safest from a microbiological standpoint: Drippings from raw meat may contain *salmonella, E. coli*, and other harmful microorganisms that might set up colonies in a wooden cutting board. Glass and other nonporous materials, washed after contact with raw meat, prevents that. At a minimum, get a board at least twelve inches by ten inches or larger. Wooden cutting boards are useful for slicing fruits and vegetables and baked goods, but most importantly as TV-food trays (for eating in the living room).

*Maintenance:* Wash with hot, soapy water to kill germs; run through the dishwasher if it fits.

*Commonly Priced at:* Starting at around $8.

## 8. MIXING BOWLS (VARIOUS SIZES)

*Primary Function:* For microwaving various foods, serving foods to guests, or just eating out of yourself.

*Look for:* Can be glass or ceramic (not metal—you want to be able to microwave with these); minimum six inches in diameter, ranging up to twelve inches or larger. Must fit inside your microwave, so measure that before you shop.

*Maintenance:* Wash after each use; they should be dishwasher-safe.

*Commonly priced at:* $12 per set and up (get at least three in different sizes, which is how many are packaged).

## 9. STIRRING SPOONS AND SPATULAS

*Primary Function:* Stirring and flipping.

*Look for:* Nonmetal (nylon, other plastics, or wood) at the end so as to not scratch nonstick utensils. Metal is OK with metal-surface frying pans.

*Maintenance:* Rinse after each use; run through the dishwasher occasionally.

*Commonly Priced at:* Under $10 each; but there are multipiece sets for $20, often with additional items you may never, ever use, such as rolling pins, whisks, and a pastry brush.

## 10. PLASTIC ORANGE-JUICE MIXER AND POTATO MASHER

*Primary Function:* Mixing and containing frozen orange and other fruit-juice concentrates.

*Look for:* The juice mixer should accommodate more than twenty-four fluid ounces and have a firm-seal lid to allow for shaking container before pouring. The potato masher is for mashing the juice concentrate; make sure it fits inside the juice container.

*Maintenance:* Must be dishwasher-safe.

*Commonly Priced at:* Approximately $10.

## 11. COLANDER

*Primary Function:* Washing vegetables, fruit, and fresh greens. Also for draining water from boiled pasta.

*Look for:* The steamer insert, cited earlier, might work for this, depending on its construction. But when entertaining, a colander will be essential if you are serving a fresh green salad and making pasta at the same time.

*Maintenance:* Dishwasher-safe. It's best to rinse the colander in between different types of food (especially after raw meat).

*Commonly Priced at:* $8 and up.

## 12. BLENDER

*Primary Function:* Chopping things really, really small and mixing food very, very fast; essential for breakfast or post-workout protein drinks.

*Look for:* The smaller versions should be fine for the single guy (recommended here primarily for fast breakfasts and protein shakes). For entertaining purposes (blending margaritas, etc.), consider the larger sizes.

*Maintenance:* Removable parts (glass or plastic) should be dishwasher-safe; you'll need to wash the electrical base part by hand.

*Commonly Priced at:* $25 and up.

## FIVE ADDITIONAL OPTIONS

### 1. GEORGE FOREMAN-STYLE GRILL

*Primary Function:* Grilling meat and vegetables fast, removing fat (the grilling surface is inclined, with grooves to channel the fat away). The beauty of these grills became clear to me the first time I made fresh salmon on one—it caramelizes the skin with signature grill marks, which enhance the sensory experience. But it's a space hog in a smaller kitchen, and I use it for only a couple of dishes (salmon, chicken, and the occasional steak or burger).

*Look for:* These come in a range of prices, the larger ones having more grilling space.

*Maintenance:* Carefully hand-wash after each use; it cannot be put in a dishwasher or immersed in a sink because of the electrical components.

*Commonly Priced at:* Ranges from $25–300.

### 2. OVEN ROASTING PAN

*Primary Function:* Baking chicken or turkey (for entertaining, or just to have lots of cooked meat on hand for leftovers). This is one of the few *A Guy's Gotta Eat* uses for the oven; be sure to remove foreign items stored there before preheating oven.

*Look for:* Large enough to accommodate a decent-sized bird. Will have a cover and rack for suspending the bird above the bottom of the pan.

*Maintenance:* Too big for the dishwasher; must be hand-scrubbed (roasting results in burned-in grease).

*Commonly Priced at:* Starting at $18.

### 3. TURBO-COOKER

*Primary Function:* Cooking multiple items (grilling meats and steaming vegetables) at the same time in a single triple-tiered utensil.

*Look for:* This concept fits the *A Guy's Gotta Eat* structure: simple (one utensil), balanced (meats and vegetables), and tasty (meat juices and aromas steam up to the vegetables, which are on a rack an inch or two over the meat). But it's also limited to that type of cooking, and doesn't allow for little vegetables (peas, husked corn, chopped broccoli), which would fall through the spaces in the grill (unless you place them on a heat-conducting plate, pan, or tinfoil).

*Maintenance:* Probably requires hand-washing.
*Commonly Priced at:* Starting at under $45.

## 4. BARBECUE GRILL

*Primary Function:* Barbecuing, a guy's favorite way to entertain.

*Look for:* What will fit in your outdoor space? Small gas-fired grills seem like a good solution, but those small tanks might last only a few meals and can run out before the meat is done, so always have a spare at the ready. Charcoal grills take time to get going and can be messy. But it's all worth it in the end, despite these obstacles.

*Maintenance:* Grills should be cleaned in between all uses. The idea that flavors are enhanced when you don't scrub the grill is offset by the insects, rodents, and microorganisms that it will draw when not in use.

*Commonly Priced at:* $30 and up.

## 5. TOASTER

*Primary Function:* Making toast, bagels, etc.

*Look for:* The classic chrome two-slicer is probably adequate (excessive bread consumption is not encouraged); chrome is good as a backup mirror.

*Maintenance:* Shake vigorously upside down to remove excess crumbs.

*Commonly Priced at:* $20 and up.

### Approximate cost of all items
Big twelve tools: $235 and up.
Five additional options: $140 and up.
Total: $375 and up.

All utensils should be washed before using to remove residue from the manufacturing, packaging, and transport processes. Study the usage instructions, fill out warranty and rebate cards—then take a step back and contemplate how smart you are already.

> Man is a tool-using animal. Without tools he is nothing, with tools he is all.
>
> —*Thomas Carlyle, philosopher*
> *1795–1881*

# 9

# a guy's gotta buy groceries (but not very often)

## A man's home is his fast-food castle

**I love that** when I need a fast snack I can make peanut butter on celery in about twelve seconds. Or microwave garbanzo beans with hot sauce and lemon juice in under a minute. When I arrive home from the gym or a run, I know I can make a chicken breast or salmon fillet in under ten minutes. After that, tubs of sweet yogurt and fruit are a fast, protein-rich dessert. I have these things all the time because I have groceries in the house.

This chapter assumes that you are like me. When we're hungry, we prefer to eat immediately. We also don't like shopping. You may have previously thought that making dinner took hours. The fact is that it doesn't. And fetching the groceries should take between thirty and ninety minutes per month—about a minute for every meal you'll make. You're going to see how one shopping trip per month will spare you wasted hours going out or calling in for food that isn't nearly as healthy as your own. The simple, mechanical act of grocery shopping will add quality to your life and probably extend it as well.

So let's go get the grub. But just as a review, here are the two guiding principles for selecting items in a grocery store:

1. *It's about Nutrition:* Almost all items will be fruit, vegetables, lean meats, low-fat dairy, or whole grains. To be avoided: processed foods, drinks listing high-fructose corn syrup among the top three ingredients, items made with refined flour (not whole grains), and high-fat, high-sugar desserts. The idea is to make smart food your only at-home option.

2. *It's about Functionality:* Most items will have a long shelf life—of between one month and two years. Some items, however—fresh greens, meats, and some dairy—will be consumed within the first fourteen days of purchase (some within three days). Food shopping can be cheaper at warehouse and large-discount retailers, where most items are sold in bulk sizes. Because almost everything you buy will have a long shelf life, the only challenge that quantity-buying presents is storage space.

When is the best time to shop? Stores get fresh goods on Wednesdays and Thursdays, so shopping close to those days gets you the best quality. Most people shop on the weekends, making for long lines. Note that the Food Marketing Institute says singles shop most often on Sundays. But perhaps that is not a smart ploy—shelf inventory of some items tends to be depleted by then and fresh produce is picked over. It just depends on what motivates you. Online shopping avoids all of this, of course. But it's a good idea to stop into a real store from time to time because you'll be more likely to try new items.

## THE GUY'S GROCERY LIST

THIS SHOPPING LIST IS divided into sections of the store to facilitate finding things according to common flow patterns. In most stores, the healthy stuff is on the periphery—fresh produce, the deli, and often frozen and refrigerated products line the outer aisles and back wall. So head your cart in that direction first. But store layouts and product-shelving systems differ, so if you get lost, quit being a guy for a minute and ask a clerk for directions.

## PRODUCE (FRESH FRUITS AND VEGETABLES)

Bananas (six to twelve)

Apples (twelve to eighteen, in two or three varieties)

Grapefruit (six to twelve)†

Limes (two to eight)†

Bulk salad greens (various types available; avoid iceberg) (one bag)*†

Red cabbage† (one to two heads)

Baby carrots (cut and peeled, pre-bagged) (two bags)†

Red onions (six to ten)

Yellow onions (one bag, or about a dozen onions)

Fresh celery† (keeps for two weeks when you slice off the base and up-end like cut flowers in a glass of water in the refrigerator)

Fresh basil*† (can be dried)

Fresh cilantro*† (can be dried)

Walnuts (shelled, one pound)

Almonds (shelled, one pound)

Other fruits and vegetables in season (summer and fall): red raspberries, blueberries, strawberries, cantaloupe*†

*Short-shelf-life goods, recommended for use within three to five days of purchase.
† Should be refrigerated.

## CONDIMENTS, SALAD DRESSINGS, AND BAKING NEEDS

Vinegar (one bottle each: red wine, apple cider, balsamic)

Salad dressings (at least four bottles; look for low-fat or fat-free in tastes that appeal to you, perhaps red-wine vinegar, Greek, Italian, Caesar, honey mustard, and ranch)

Sugar or sweetener (Equal, NatraTaste, Splenda, and others)

Cooking spray (olive oil and butter varieties)

Olive oil (other choices: flaxseed, canola, peanut, and grapeseed)

Tomato sauce (four jars or cans, minimum; try several varieties)

Mayonnaise (one jar; try low-fat or fat-free varieties)

Raisins (one to two twenty-four-ounce cans, may be in the snack section)

Salt

Pepper

Cinnamon

Oregano (dried)

Pre-mixed spices (two to four varieties of your choice)

Lemon juice

Prepared mustard

Horseradish

Parmesan or Romano cheese, grated (one canister)

Minced garlic

Hot sauce/Tabasco

Steak sauce

## BEVERAGES AND JUICES

Frozen orange juice (frozen because it's more space efficient; one twelve-ounce container lasts four days); substitutes are other citrus-based drinks (grapefruit juice, lemon-lime juice, or cranberry juice, but be careful of cocktail varieties, which contain a lot of sugar)

Suggestion: Green tea (strongly associated with reduced risks of several types of cancer)

Avoid juices and drinks that list "high-fructose corn syrup" among the first few ingredients (which means the drink is essentially sugar and water)

## GRAINS, CEREALS, AND BREADS

Oatmeal, unsweetened (two to four forty-two ounce canisters; individual packs in flavored varieties often have added sugar and are more expensive ounce for ounce)

One loaf of whole-grain bread ("wheat" bread is not always whole grain; look for the word "whole" preceding the grain list in the ingredients)

Brown rice, instant (one to two boxes, approximately fourteen ounces; perfectly acceptable alternatives are other varieties of wild rice)

Whole-grain or spinach pasta (one to two bags)

# HFCS

**F**ARMERS WORRY THEIR kids might smoke corn silk, but the more common high is from HFCS–high-fructose corn syrup–pumped into everything from soda and juice drinks to ketchup, tomato sauce, salad dressing, baked desserts, applesauce, dry cereal, ice cream, and maple syrup (you thought it came from trees in Vermont?).

HFCS is a processed sugar, so it is digested and absorbed quickly, forcing your pancreas to pump out insulin in rapid response–the physiological reaction to the consumption of all processed carbohydrates. In heavy use by the food industry since the early 1970s (when it was found to be a cheaper and more versatile sweetener than cane and sugar beets) many dietitians believe HFCS to be the most heinous culprit in the fattening of America.

Rule of thumb: Avoid foods that list HFCS or "high-fructose corn syrup" in the ingredient label. Some brands of tomato sauce contain it, while others do not. Other words to avoid as primary ingredients include sugar, honey, fruit juice concentrate, and molasses. Alternatively, milk, plain yogurt, and 100 per cent fruit juice contain only naturally occurring sugar–and along with it carry many other beneficial nutrients.

## BEANS AND OTHER CANNED GOODS

Black beans (four to ten cans)
Red kidney beans (four to ten cans)
Garbanzo beans, a.k.a. cece beans, chickpeas (four to ten cans)
Stewed tomatoes, regular or Italian -tyle (six to twelve cans)
Tuna fish, solid fancy or white albacore in water (four to twelve cans)
Salmon (one to two cans)
Chicken (two to four cans)
Salsa (two to four jars, any variety)
Pickled herring in red wine sauce (one jar, just to try it)
Sardines (one can, just to try it)
Anchovies (only you know if you like them)
Peanut butter (one jar, regular or chunky; all-natural is better because it has less sugar and no hydrogenated oils)
Beef broth (one to two cans)
Chicken broth (one to two cans)
Pre-made soups (for very lazy days; broth, not creamy varieties; check

differences in nutrition facts as they may be high in sodium, a concern for people with high blood pressure)

## FROZEN FOODS (MEATS, VEGETABLES, AND FRUIT)

Boneless, skinless chicken breasts (one to three 2.5-pound or larger bags; also sold in boxes)

Broccoli spears (two to four boxes/bags)

Chopped broccoli (two to four boxes/bags)

Corn (two to four boxes/bags)

Peas (two to four boxes/bags)

Green peppers (two to four boxes/bags)

Cauliflower (two to four boxes/bags)

Green beans (two to four boxes/bags)

Spinach (two to four boxes/bags)

Edamame (soybeans in the pod, one bag)

Mixed medley: carrots, cauliflower, broccoli (two to four boxes/bags)

Raspberries (one bag)

Blueberries (one bag)

Strawberries (one bag)

All other available frozen fruits and vegetables that appeal to you, such as brussels sprouts, asparagus, squash, zucchini, or lima beans

Keep in mind that these will all have to fit into your freezer, along with frozen orange juice concentrate, chicken, and other meats. With efficient packing, I can fit approximately forty boxes and bags of vegetables, along with twelve containers of orange juice concentrate, four bags of chicken breasts, and three or four miscellaneous packages (my freezer capacity is 4.8 cubic feet, a standard size).

## FRESH LEAN MEATS AND FISH

Ground turkey, approximately 93 percent lean (one to two packs, approximately one pound each)*

Salmon fillets (under one pound)*

Lean red meat*: Choose four to eight portions (one portion: approximately four ounces) from the following list of leanest cuts (there are other lean cuts of beef, pork, and even lamb, but these are the easiest to prepare):

Top sirloin steak

Top loin steak

Tenderloin steak
T-bone steak
Ground beef (95 percent lean)

*Must be consumed within three days, or frozen for up to six months. Since you won't be able to consume all of this, purchase some frozen meat or fish where available (frozen is often, but not always, cheaper per pound). Also, beware of ground turkey that is less than 85-percent lean; likely, the skin was ground into the mix.

## DAIRY

Fat-free/low-fat (1 percent) cottage cheese (two to four sixteen-ounce tubs)
Fat-free/low-fat yogurt (four to six thirty-two-ounce tubs; plain or vanilla, can be sugar-free)
Liquid eggs (two to six items, sold in eight- and sixteen-ounce portions). Get two kinds: egg whites (100 percent liquid egg whites) for use in protein drinks, and egg substitutes, also made with egg whites, but with added ingredients that include yellow coloring (for non-drink uses)
Traditional eggs (one dozen)
Butter (not margarine due to hydrogenation; smallest quantity available)

## PAPER PRODUCTS/WRAPS

Film (saran) wrap (one roll)
Zipper-style sandwich bags (large and small)
Paper towels (two to four rolls)
Tinfoil (one roll)
While they have very little to do with nutrition and eating, other things you might pick up at a grocery store include bathroom tissue, cleaning supplies, and dental, shaving, and other grooming products.

**Approximate cost for all groceries: $320***
*Based on prices in the Chicago area, December 2002.
*Note: Several items will last for months, so subsequent trips to the grocery store will likely cost less.

# HOW TO READ NUTRITION FACTS ON FOOD LABELS

**T**HE FOOD AND Drug Administration standardized how major nutrients and ingredients are represented on food packaging by introducing the Nutrition Facts label in the early 1990s. Since that introduction, consumer studies found these labels are effective for individuals who are motivated to address health and weight-management issues.

The following are the components to the Nutrition Facts label:

**Servings per container.** Get a relative sense of how much of everything is in the entire package—if you sneak over to the ice cream case, note how a pint is *four* servings.

**Total fat and types (in grams).** Look to see how much of the fat is saturated versus other types of fat (unsaturated, mono- and polyunsaturated). In general, you want less of the saturated, more of the unsaturated, with mono- and polyunsaturated as the middle ground. Trans fats, to be avoided, will be recorded on all food labels by 2006.

**Protein (grams).** If you want a higher-protein meal, this is a key number.

**Ratio of protein to fat.** Strive for a protein-to-fat ratio of 3:1 or greater, but note that certain healthy items (salmon, peanut butter, nuts, olive oil) will fare poorly in this analysis because their values come from omega-3 fatty acids, vitamin E, and other antioxidants rather than a favorable protein-to-fat ratio.

**Ingredients:** This list helps you understand if the sources are close to nature or much removed via processing. Ingredients are listed according to percent of composition of the whole product, from largest to smallest. Words to look out for: bleached flour, refined flour, high-fructose corn syrup, hydrogenated vegetable oil.

Exempt from current nutrition labeling laws are fresh produce and fresh meats because of the variability in stock and size. In restaurants, only fast-food menus are subject to published nutrition information (available from in-store brochures, signs, and on company Web sites). Casual and fine-dining establishments are exempt because of portion and stock variability; only when a health claim is made, such as "heart-healthy Southwestern chicken," is the establishment required to provide the nutrition facts to support it.

## INVENTORY MANAGEMENT

WHILE MOST OF WHAT you've purchased has a long shelf life, the refrigerated items and some dry goods (such as oatmeal) will spoil or have bugs that appear magically over time. The quantities in the above list are purposefully smaller than what you might consume in a month; I kept it to a conservative amount simply to reduce waste with items you may not like. If an item gets used quickly, that's a clear indication you should purchase more on your next shopping trip.

In subsequent shopping trips, you'll bring home items that may not yet be depleted on your shelves. Rotate your inventory: move items from left to right, back to front, and top to bottom (or some other system you devise) when you bring in new stock such that cans, bags, or boxes do not linger in a back corner past their "use by" or "best if purchased by" dates.

## YOUR FIRST DINNER

OK, YOU ARE HOME and stocked. Are you hungry? You're not going to order in tonight. Here are two simple, satisfying meals the tired shopper can make in less than fifteen minutes:

### #1 Chicken Broccoli Express

**You need:**

✎One microwavable bowl, large enough to hold all the ingredients

Two chicken breasts (one would work just as well)

¼-inch splash of lemon juice

One bag/box of broccoli (chopped or spears)

Salt and pepper to taste (as much as you like)

Parmesan cheese (optional)

Optional: about twenty drops (a drizzle) of olive oil

**Preparation:**

1. Put both chicken breasts, side by side, in bowl. Add lemon juice; use a drizzle of olive oil (optional). Add salt, pepper, and oregano to taste. Cover loosely with paper towels (to hold in steam).
2. Microwave on high for four to six minutes (reduce cook times by about one-third overall if using only one breast); time varies by relative strength of microwave oven.

3. Flip breasts over. Add bag/box of broccoli to same bowl, on top of chicken.

4. Microwave on high for another two to four minutes. Stir vegetables.

5. Microwave on high for another two to four minutes. Leave standing a minute or two to steam. Slice one breast in half to see if it's cooked through (with no pink meat in the center); if not, slice the chicken into bite-sized pieces and microwave on high for another minute or two.

Eat from the bowl you made it in. Sprinkle with Parmesan cheese to taste.

## #2 Salmon and Onions

**You need:**
🔨 One skillet
One fillet of salmon
¼-inch splash of lemon juice
One yellow or red onion (chopped or sliced into rings)
Half a can of diced tomatoes
Salt and pepper to taste (as much as you like)

**Preparation:**
1. Put salmon in skillet (no oil necessary; the fish has its own oil).
2. Chop onion.
3. Turn oven burner to medium-high and move the fish around to oil up the surface of the skillet.
4. Add lemon juice, then salt and pepper to taste.
5. Add chopped onion and half-can of diced tomatoes. Cover skillet.
6. After about three to four minutes (a little more if the fish was frozen), use a spatula or wooden spoon to stir the onions and flip the fish over.
7. Cook another three to four minutes, turning the heat to high. You want the fish and vegetables to be crisp but not burned.

As you savor the fish, allow yourself the satisfaction that this particular meal lowers your chance of having a heart attack this month (see page 254 for details). You've also won the first and perhaps most decisive battle to take back the plate. Congratulations.

# PART III

# GET TO WORK

## GUYS COOKING

fall into two categories: engineers and artists. The engineers work well with instructions and precise amounts. They follow directions. They need a plan, and they don't like change. They worry about structural integrity but may lack an intuitive sense. They like the outcome to meet their expectations.

Artists go by feel. They abhor confining directions. They might work with a general plan, but always break from convention. They may see a structure in things, but sniff out opportunities for enhancement and innovation. Not unlike Pollock or

Kandinsky, they find meaning where others see chaos. The artist is willing to risk disaster.

Not everyone is an artist. Hence, meal preparation in the following chapters follows specific instructions. You might even call them recipes. But if you're the kind of guy who goes about things by feel, don't feel confined to exact amounts or only the ingredients listed. You should feel comfortable about making substitutions—use cottage cheese when you're out of yogurt, for example—because it's far better that you make something at home instead of ordering fast food.

Taste is personal, after all. Start by identifying what you like and what you will look forward to eating at the end of the day, on a lazy weekend for lunch, or every morning for breakfast. Over time you should gain the confidence to improvise on your main meal components.

To get started, kick off your shoes, pop something funny into the DVD player, and crack open a pilsner. Find your *flow*, baby. In time, you can learn to create smart dishes that are uniquely you.

# 10

# a guy's gotta master a few basics in the kitchen

## Rules of thumb for cooking

**The first-time** cook is vulnerable to disaster and failure. But food is much less complicated than ready-to-assemble furniture or the IRS 1040-EZ form. Some basic instruction and a little experience will bring success for years to come. I cite my own fiascos from unschooled attempts at meal making: a gray microwaved steak, peas overcooked to the point where the green was gone and burnt, blackened tomato sauce. These experiences could have dissuaded me from cooking altogether had I not also stumbled into a few good meals, largely by accident. If your own experiences with cooking are bad, take heart. It's not rocket science. Nor is there a gene that dooms you to failure. You just need a few pointers. Your confidence in the kitchen will grow when you understand how food works and how to create satisfying meals.

We are lucky to live in a time when modern equipment reduces the opportunity for error. Our great-grandmothers, for example, would have killed for nonstick pans. Commercially prepared sauces, dressings, and spices cut out steps and deliver taste consistency. And while the microwave is no place for expensive cuts of red meat, it vastly improves our ability to make fast meals with minimum clean-up—for example, chicken and fish nuke well with a little lemon juice and salt, flipped at the midpoint and covered with a paper towel to hold in the moisture.

As a general guide, a complete meal (often but not always contained within a single dish) boils down to three primary components:

⊃ *Main Stuff:* The heart of the meal, which ranges from chicken breasts to kidney beans, tuna, grilled steaks, eggs, peanuts, protein powder, and yogurt.

⊃ *Crunch:* Vegetables, nuts, and fruit, such as celery, walnuts, and apples in salads, soups, and casseroles. Broadly defined, Crunch is about texture, such as the grain of pumpernickel, the wet, crisp break of lettuce, or even the creamy smoothness of yogurt. Sometimes, the Crunch component is already present in Main Stuff, but more is more when it comes to Crunch. Just think of what your teeth cut through in a great deli sandwich.

⊃ *Flavor:* Everything from chapter 7, including citric juice (lemon and lime), vinegar (balsamic and others), hot sauce, oregano, salt and pepper, sweetener, Parmesan and Romano cheeses (grated), prepared salad dressing (lower-fat versions), olive oil, onions and garlic, cilantro, mustards, horseradish, steak sauce, prepared spice blends (in dry packs), cinnamon, spicy garden mix, ginger root, minced garlic, sun-dried tomatoes, basil, salsa, and about five hundred other things. Additionally, flavors arise from the foods themselves, meat in particular; cooking causes some juices to drip to the bottom of the cooking utensil, which can be retrieved (scraped or deglazed) and dripped onto the dish. Cooked cabbage (a dependably crunchy vegetable) might not be so great until you mix in microwaved chicken (for protein), celery and onions (more crunch), and the chicken juices with extra lemon and cilantro (flavor).

If you're a beginner cook and you're making your first meals at home but don't have a particular dish in mind, you might just scan your cupboards, refrigerator, and freezer for these three components. With experience, this part of meal preparation becomes intuitive—and will take all of ten seconds to accomplish.

## COOKING RISK MANAGEMENT

THE NEW GUY to the kitchen must accept a certain degree of risk. As with all new ventures in life, you will do better when you mitigate that risk with plans and tactics—such as the following basic rules of thumb for subsistence-level cooking:

**THINK IT THROUGH:** When you decide what you want to make, assess the ingredients, tools, and process needed to make it happen. Mentally map out how you'll cook frozen ground beef, for example, with a bag of corn, a can of diced tomatoes, a chopped onion, and other ingredients. The meat will take longer to cook; adding the other ingredients at the midpoint prevents overcooking of the vegetables. This is pretty simple when you are making a one-dish meal for yourself, a bit more complex when you are entertaining and making several dishes. Sketching out a plan on paper is a pretty smart approach.

**VARY COLORS:** We also eat with our eyes, appreciating on a sensory level a mix of such foods as cooked meat and brightly colored vegetables. But aesthetics play a physiological role, too: A variety of colors tells us the food has nutrient balance, variety, and moderation. The fact that we react favorably to color variation may be a result of evolution or simply learned conditioning, but the outcome is the same. Sure, the fiber and vitamins in green lettuce are great, but you need other vitamins and protein from beans, meat, and dairy—which is why you make a salad with all those other things added.

**DON'T KILL YOURSELF WITH BAD MEAT:** Meat must be adequately cooked so you don't die or get horrible intestinal problems from it. In general, food must be cooked at temperatures high and long enough to kill harmful microorganisms, such as *salmonella* and *E. coli.* Safe storage of leftovers and reheating are part of this equation. For more on navigating some inherent dangers of food, see "Avoiding Leftover Sickness" on page 179 in chapter 11. Fortunately, the more complicated concerns about uncooked meat in the home have to do with roasts, such as the holiday turkey. Most recipes in this book involve thinner cuts of meat for which undercooking is both easy to visually spot and unlikely to happen.

**UNDERSTAND HEAT:** Those dials on your stove are pretty important. The natural instinct for many guys is to always set the oven to "high" because, duh, it will cook dinner faster. Well, not exactly. That's a quick way to burn things on the outside without cooking the inside—frozen ground sirloin or chicken breasts, for example. Here are the basic cooking levels and their purpose:

⊃ Lo/Low is for slow cooking, or most often for keeping something warm after it's been cooked. The food itself should be at or above 140°F, higher than what bacteria can tolerate (medium-rare meat cooks at around 145°F, well done at 170°F); to achieve these food temperatures, you need to set the stove-top temperature higher than that—around 275°F—because some heat is lost to the surrounding area (the air, stove top, and utensils). Many stove settings do not provide temperature readings; hand-held temperature gauges can provide assurance to exacting types.

⊃ Medium (350°F and/or medium flame on a gas stove top) is also a slower cooking setting, a bit faster than Lo/Low. It is best when used with meats and other products that come in frozen blocks. When cooking frozen ground beef that you neglected to thaw in advance, use a spatula to shave off the thawed parts to more evenly cook the meat.

⊃ Medium-High (425°F and/or medium-high flame on a gas stove top) is your most frequently used temperature. It is pretty fast but requires attention; stir and flip the food so it heats evenly. Frozen chicken breasts can be cooked at this temperature, but always slice one in half to make sure it's white (not pink) all the way through.

⊃ High (450–500°F and/or as high as the flame goes on a gas stove top) is for boiling water and browning things, such as chopped onions and meat that's already cooked (at Medium-High). Use with caution—heat can make food spit fat.

**DON'T OVERCOOK VEGETABLES:** Nature gives us fresh, firm, crisp, and beautiful vegetables. Some cooking brings out flavors (e.g., in cauliflower and broccoli) that certainly make them taste better. But subjecting vegetables to too much cooking can destroy nutrients and make them taste, feel, and look bland. In one-pot dishes where all the ingredients cook together, the vegetables usually are added at a late stage to minimize overcooking. Steaming vegetables beats immersion in boiling water, which tends to leach nutrients faster.

**A LITTLE OIL MAKES EVERYTHING WORK BETTER:** Olive oil not only helps conduct heat to food from pots and pans and prevents sticking, it also serves as a catalyst for other dietary nutrients within the body and contributes to a feeling of fullness. Oil is composed of fat, and despite bad press over the years, anywhere between 20 and 40 percent of our calories should come from this macronutrient (bodybuilders and advocates of the Pritikin diet would dip as low as 10 percent, but neither are realistic over the long term). The point is to use plant-based fats (olive, peanut, canola, and flaxseed oils are good options) because these are highest in healthier monounsaturated and polyunsaturated fats (versus unhealthy saturated fats). Because you'll get a heavier dose of fat in the meals you eat outside of the home, it makes sense to add only a little oil when doing your own cooking.

**MOST STUFF FROM CANS AND JARS IS READY TO EAT:** Think about all the major canned foods—tuna, beans, stewed tomatoes, soup stock, applesauce, and tomato sauce, just to name a few. Each of them is safe to eat out of the can or jar—sometimes I drink the applesauce from its container to save on dishwashing (not recommended over eating actual apples, by the way). Foods in cans and jars are cooked or pasteurized in processing, which kills the germs. (Canned salmon might also qualify, but I can't wrap my tongue around that one: Salmon needs a hot, crispy outer layer—see chapter 13 for one approach.) Here's the beauty of it: Most of these foods are just a few minutes away from being on your dinner plate.

**EXPERIMENTATION IS GOOD:** Cooking is more art than science (*baking* is science, and thank God this book has nothing to do with making cakes). When trying something new, add conservative amounts of the item to a small portion of the dish; adjust taste from there. Tinkering with the various components of foods and recipes is how you can find the most satisfaction when making food for yourself.

**GOOGLE GOURMET:** Bored and out of ideas? Or maybe you have ideas but want a little advice? Use the Internet's most helpful search engine, Google.com, to find new ways to use ingredients. Just input some key ingredients (for example, chicken and sauerkraut) plus the word "recipe" and in the time it takes to say "bandwidth," you should have a lot of choices. We live in an enchanted age.

**MEASURING THINGS:** With a modest amount of cooking experience you will measure nothing. But you have to work within some ranges, especially as a beginner. You could go out and purchase kitchen measuring instruments (a measuring cup and spoons)—for the engineer types, this may provide a certain confidence when working in a kitchen. But very specific measurements suggest a level of precision that just isn't necessary in cooking. The instructions in this chapter assume you didn't purchase measuring spoons and cups; instead we bring you a Guy's Measuring System, as follows:

⊃ *Cup:* Just use a standard coffee cup, about eight ounces (not a tankard mug and not a demitasse teacup, which chances are you do not have sitting around the house anyway). Measure the cup once and you will have a reference point forever. A cup and a half would be a tall, thin drinking glass.

⊃ *Large Spoon:* A soup spoon, roughly equivalent to a standard tablespoon; whether it's heaping or level is up to you. But not a serving spoon. A lot of guys think the extra-large spoons used to serve things from dishes onto plates are tablespoons. They are mistaken. The size of spoon we're talking about here is the kind you would use to eat soup, not the one for transferring soup from pot to bowl.

⊃ *Small Spoon:* The smaller kind of spoon, quite often the equivalent of the official teaspoon.

⊃ *Glop:* A heaping, large soup-spoon quantity.

⊃ *Dollop:* A glop of something semi-solid, like peanut butter or yogurt.

⊃ *Dash:* Take the bottle (of vinegar, lemon juice, or whatever) and momentarily tip it—for about half a second—into the food. A bartender does this with cocktail ingredients such as benedictine, grenadine, or bitters.

⊃ *Jigger:* To get something completely wet with the ingredient by holding it over the dish a moment or two longer than a dash. For example, a jigger of salad dressing on chicken breasts. In bartender parlance, a jigger is approximately equivalent to the amount of liquid in a shot glass; the engineering type might use a shot glass if he prefers.

**KNOW YOUR COOKING ACTION VERBS:** All skills require short-cut terms, and cooking has its own set of them. Here are a few basics to make you more conversant in the language of meal preparation.

⊃ *Stir-fry:* This is when you cook stuff in a small amount of oil; the end result is that you brown or "caramelize" parts of a meal. Some call it sautéing but we won't; most French words are necessary only to the pretentious. Place onions, garlic, or other vegetables in a light amount of olive oil in a skillet, usually for five or ten minutes before adding a Main Stuff ingredient, such as a breast of chicken.

⊃ *Deglaze:* This could be called making gravy, except you use a little bit of wine instead of cornstarch. This is when you pour some old wine into a pan that was used to stir-fry chicken, beef, or other meats. The leftover fat and other natural juices, cooked for about thirty seconds with the wine, will become a tasty dressing to pour over the meat or vegetables.

➲ *Searing:* This is cooking in a flash of heat, such as putting a T-bone steak in an oiled pan already at a high temperature. It fuses in the natural juices, which makes for a juicier meal. Once seared and sealed, you can continue cooking at a reduced temperature to achieve rare, medium, or well-done meat.

➲ *Simmer:* Cooking food at a temperature setting just below a full boil, in the medium-high stove setting. It mixes flavors and tastes to produce a tasty end product.

➲ *Denature or Tenderize:* Exposing meats to acidic juices or spices to break down the muscle fiber, resulting in more tender meat. For example, soaking cuts of sirloin or other meat in Italian dressing prior to barbecuing.

➲ *Mince:* Chopping something into teeny, tiny pieces. Especially done with garlic and herbs.

➲ *Cube:* Just like it sounds, you are cutting things into cube-like shapes, usually creating bite-size pieces. Done with meats and tuberous vegetables (sweet potatoes, for example). This is done for the convenience of the eater—there is no need for a knife while eating cubed chicken, for example—or to speed cooking (cubed sweet potatoes cook more evenly and quickly than when cooked whole).

There are many other terms from the lexicon of cooking, but on a basic level you don't need to know them.

Cooking is not foolproof, but there's a lot of forgiveness in food. An extra dash or two of most ingredients won't ruin the dish—it'll just make it taste more like the ingredient you're adding. After all, taste is personal.

# a guy's gotta make a meal in less than fifteen minutes

## Subsistence cooking for the beginner

**The promise is** simple. You can make a breakfast, lunch, dinner, snack, or dessert in less than a third of the time required for a pizza delivery—some meals and snacks are faster than reheating a leftover slice.

This chapter provides the directions—in some cases, full-fledged recipes, but with many items it's just a matter of mixing and microwaving. For guys who are new to the game, scan the following pages and try the things that look easiest to you. Build up your confidence, then move on to something a little more challenging.

## THE DISHES

WE LIVE IN a world of conformists. Breakfast is in the morning, lunch at noon, and dinner sometime after five. But I know people who eat Cheerios for dinner, while some others eat beans at breakfast. Meals here are arranged according to American traditions. Don't let that stop you from eating peas in the morning and eggs at night.

### BREAKFAST

Let's assess the relative time factors of mornings. For most guys, no time means no breakfast or a bad breakfast. Bad breakfasts are found at drive-throughs, convenience stores, coffeehouses, muffin kiosks, or morning meetings. Not much good can come from any of these places. So if you're serious about this whole thing, it makes complete sense that you give it some effort—and time. But not very much time: Unless you're a business road warrior or live in a van down by the river, this is a meal where proximity to a kitchen is all but guaranteed.

But doesn't a guy cut calories and fat by skipping breakfast entirely? Aside from how a good breakfast averts the 10:30 A.M. donut, there is an important physiological component. Every time we eat and digest something (meals as well as snacks) our metabolism is revved up through what's called the thermal effect of food (TEF). When we regularly skip meals—periods without eating for around five or more hours—our metabolism slows down because it perceives starvation. This ultimately leads to the body expending fewer calories, counter to most peoples' intended effect of weight management or loss. Again, this relates back to our species' caveman condition, where the body efficiently stored energy (fat) when a food shortage occurred. The bottom line is: *Don't skip breakfast.*

Breakfast items are organized by ascending degrees of difficulty and time commitment—Simple, followed by Cereals, then Eggs, Dude. Find what fits you and your morning routines.

#### Simple

Making each of these should take between thirty seconds and five minutes. Many fit in to-go coffee containers for in-car dining (not recommended from a safety standpoint).

### Protein Bars

This is by far the easiest and wimpiest approach you can take to breakfast. But if a bar's nutrition facts offer a protein-to-fat ratio of 3:1 or greater per serving, it's a far better choice than hash browns, sausage, and certainly donuts. The growing popularity of protein bars might be due to their nutritional value. But let's be honest, they have improved considerably in recent years and they now taste and chew like candy bars. Nothin' much wrong with that. Look for varieties that have 200 to 250 calories or fewer per bar. Eat just one—and chase it with an apple or orange for its fiber, antioxidants, and ability to freshen your breath.

### Yogurt and Fruit

From your shopping trip, you have large tubs of low-fat or fat-free yogurt (usually, these have a favorable protein-to-fat ratio). Take one whole piece of fruit—or more, if you like—put it in a bowl, and pour yogurt all over the top. Sprinkle cinnamon on top, if desired. Add wheat germ or flaxseeds, if so inclined. Protein, fructose, fiber, and antioxidants constitute a great morning meal.

The best morning fruits are: bananas, apple slices, pear slices, oranges, grapefruit, raisins, grapes, and berries. In fact, I can't think of a fruit that's bad in the morning. In a pinch, substitute "no sugar added" fruit preserves (jam) or canned fruit; most have a good dose of added refined sugar, so just be wary of that (it's still better to get sugar-added fruit than a 380-calorie, 19-fat-gram blueberry muffin).

### Yogurt, Peanut Butter, and Fruit

Nuke a glob or two of peanut butter in a bowl. When it's soupy/drippy, dump about three times as much yogurt on top. Add fruit, mix, and eat. Substitute nuts (walnuts, almonds, or peanuts—about a handful) for peanut butter, if desired.

### Protein Egg Shakes (No Blender)

In a large container (recycled twenty-six-ounce tomato sauce jars are exceptionally good for this), combine orange juice and pasteurized egg whites. Stir vigorously, then drink. This works slightly better with a blender, but then you have to deal with washing it. This non-blender method helps develop the forearms.

### Protein Shakes (with Blender)

Go on a blender bender. About a fifth of the people we surveyed—guys who routinely work out and eat sensibly—make their breakfasts in a blender (a few guys even make their own smoothies at lunch). Reasons vary; for some it's convenience, for others it's a way to achieve nutritional balance. Smart blender breakfasts have three components:

1. *Protein:* A combination of dairy (skim milk, low-fat yogurt, or cottage cheese) or soy substitute (soy milk, preferred by people who are lactose-intolerant), pasteurized eggs (egg whites sold in cartons don't require cooking), and/or protein powder.
2. *Fruit or fruit juice:* Almost any will do. But only fruit *juice*, not fruit *drink*, which is made of high-fructose corn syrup instead of 100 percent fruit.
3. *Ice:* Chills it and creates a texture.

Combine varying amounts of the above per taste and pay attention to the total amount of calories, fat, and protein in the final product (read the labels and consult the list of fruit calories beginning on page 44 for reference). Use your imagination and try to at least change the fruit from day to day. Five suggestions (supplemented with protein powder, if you prefer, and ice):

1. Cottage cheese and blueberries
2. Yogurt, orange juice, and chopped walnuts
3. Skim milk and strawberries
4. Egg whites, orange juice, and raspberries
5. Skim milk, a spoonful of peanut butter, and a large apple

### Toast Meals

Whole-grain bread toasted with a little butter is a good start, but you'll need some added protein to successfully carry you through the morning—and make it less likely you'll go to the muffin kiosk or the deadly donut shop. Two suggestions: Have a stash of hard-boiled eggs ready. Peel and slice, put on buttered toast. Carry one or two eggs in your pocket for eating later in the morning (but eat it within two hours of removing it from the refrigerator). Options include lower-fat mozzarella cheese, a handful of nuts, or peanut butter. But enough's enough on the peanut butter. A glob or two in a day, no more than six globs each week.

# FIVE-MINUTE WONDERS

**H**UNGRY AND IN a hurry? The quick answer is right at home for guys smart enough to stock up on basic groceries. Try these six basic meals:

### Eggs anytime

Mix eggs or egg substitutes with frozen vegetables and/or a chopped onion and a preferred spice in a skillet or an oiled microwaveable bowl. Few foods hold off hunger as well as eggs—nothing says you can't eat them for lunch or dinner.

### Blender drinks

Combine any dairy product (yogurt, cottage cheese, or skim milk) with fruit, fruit juice, ice, and sweetener (if desired). Blend and drink (making sure to rinse the glass pitcher to avoid a difficult clean-up later).

### Beans and . . .

Almost anything goes with mashed-up beans. For starters, take a can of garbanzo beans, mash with a fork in a bowl, then add Tabasco and lemon juice. A little cheese, anything green, and even some raisins can make this even more interesting.

### Yogurt and . . .

Faster than using a blender and with less clean-up. Just start tossing fruit into sweetened yogurt for a meal that tastes like a dessert. With plain yogurt your options are even greater—canned tomatoes (drained) with pepper and chopped-up pepperoncinis gives you a spicy meal.

### Cottage cheese and . . .

See yogurt, above.

### Soup

This requires less than three minutes of work but requires another ten minutes on the stove (on medium-high heat) before your first spoonful. But it's easy. In a skillet, simply combine one can of soup broth and an equal amount of water, a bag of frozen mixed vegetables (peas, broccoli, cauliflower), and a can each of tomatoes and beans. Spice to taste. Or skip the stove: You can make the same thing in a large microwavable bowl in about the same amount of time (times vary by microwave strength).

### Cereals

#### Ready-Made and Cold

There are whole-grain cereals, and there are all the rest. Only whole grains will do; don't even think about the kind that comes in pastel or chocolate colors, or has an animated character as a spokesfigure. The most popular whole-grain cereals and 100-percent-bran products include Shredded Wheat, Grape Nuts, Wheaties, Wheat Chex, All Bran, 100% Bran, Cheerios, and Nutri-Grain. But even with whole grains and low-fat milk or yogurt, you might raise the protein content a bit with a protein-powder supplement to avert hunger in late morning.

#### Oatmeal

This is my breakfast. The FDA allows Quaker Oats to claim that oatmeal lowers cholesterol and contributes to overall cardiovascular health. On their own, oats don't have a whole lot of taste, but they are sticky; I remember that as a kid we used oatmeal in art projects. But it's also a great medium for the tasty things I put in my (large) bowl of oatmeal:

Protein powder* (one scoop or less)
Fruit (raisins, chopped apples, bananas, berries in season)* (one cup total)
Chopped nuts** (one to two large tablespoons)
Cinnamon**
Non-fat yogurt (added after cooking)* (one dollop)

*Always added
**Sometimes added (note that high-calorie additions such as nuts are recommended only for individuals engaged in regular exercise programs. As a rule of thumb, use only two protein sources per meal, such as protein powder and yogurt, or nuts and yogurt)

Making this takes me about three minutes to gather the ingredients, chop whatever needs chopping, and mix all of it. Then I put it in the microwave for five minutes, during which time I jump in the shower. By the time I'm clean, my oatmeal is ready.

#### Eggs, Dude

"Studies show that high-protein foods such as eggs have a dampening effect on hunger, whereas high-carbohydrate breakfasts can leave you hungry by 10:00 A.M.," says Donald J. McNamara, Ph.D.

Well, just to qualify his statement, McNamara is executive director of the Egg Nutrition Center in Washington, D.C. His job is to hawk eggs. But what he says is true: the seven to ten grams of protein (with four to five grams of fat, only a third of it saturated) in each egg does have its holding power. And they are almost universally appealing.

Nature was pretty clever when she made eggs. The yolk has all the fat in it (with some of the egg's protein and all of its cholesterol), while egg whites (albumen) are pure protein. You can separate the two from each other yourself, if you wish to have a no-fat protein meal, but commercial brands of egg whites and egg substitutes are plentiful and easy to use. The recipes presented here can be made with whole eggs or egg whites.

# HOW TO HARD-BOIL EGGS

**E**GGS ARE SMART nutrition—with complete protein, satiating fat, and virtually no carbohydrates—and they're also pretty versatile. Good from the griddle, the hard-boiled version is also great out of your pocket. Only the banana has it beat on its own resilient packaging. It's also a good food you can make ahead of time, and hard-boiled eggs can last up to a week or two. But there are tricks to cooking hard-boiled eggs safely and so that their shells peel off easily. This advice from the Georgia Egg Commission:

1. Place eggs in single layer in saucepan. Add enough tap water to rise at least one inch above eggs.
2. Cover and quickly bring just to boiling. Turn off heat.
3. If necessary, remove pan from burner to prevent further boiling. Let eggs stand, covered, in the hot water about fifteen to seventeen minutes for large eggs (adjust time up or down for each size larger or smaller).
4. Immediately run cold water over eggs or place them in ice water until completely cooled.
5. To remove shell, crack it by tapping gently all over. Roll egg between hands to loosen shell, then peel, starting at large end (that's where the air bubble is). Hold egg under running cold water to help ease off shell.

### Nuclear Egg

Perhaps the simplest yet most technologically advanced way to make a quick egg breakfast is by cracking one or two eggs into a bowl and microwaving them for about forty-five seconds. Low-fat cheese on top works too. Some bowls would need a spritz of cooking spray, and some people need to eat this on a piece of whole-wheat bread or English muffin. It also makes a smart snack any time of the day.

### Eggs in the Pan

From start to finish, most fried-egg dishes can be made in around fifteen minutes. The egg part is easy. Coat a pan with cooking spray, set the stove to medium-high, set the eggs loose, and either flip them when hard or scramble them with a spatula while cooking. The frying part is done in about three minutes. With a microwave and commercial egg substitutes, it's about the same amount of time.

But to make it a little more interesting and nutritionally diverse, enter omelet and frittata territory. The difference between omelets and frittatas is largely aesthetic, in my opinion. An omelet is a little harder to make in that you have to hold it all together in a neat little fold. A frittata, loosely defined, is an egg mess: everything cooked up and in a pile—no flipping or folding involved. The omelet almost always has cheese, vegetables, and spices in it; the frittata can, too. My experience with omelets is that you have to be careful about portion sizes and overall proportion. If it gets too big, it falls apart—leaving you with a frittata. So why start the day with a failure? Every greasy diner in the free world serves omelets anyway—master the frittata at home.

Note that if your goal is to lose weight by reducing calories and fat while increasing your protein intake, egg substitutes provide significant advantages: One whole egg has about 70-80 calories, and has 4.5 grams of fat and 5 grams of protein. Egg substitutes vary a bit by brand, but three portions, at a physical bulk of three times that of an egg (140 grams), can have 75 calories, with no fat and 15 grams of protein.

# Broccoli Tomato Frittata

It's a great, crunchy meal that helps you start the day out right.

### You need:

Skillet and spatula

Cooking spray

Eggs (four, or one eight-ounce carton of egg whites/egg substitute)

Chopped broccoli (one bag of frozen)

Tomatoes (one can of stewed)

Small onion, chopped

Optional: Cheese (one handful, grated—low-fat cheddar, mozzarella, feta, or Swiss)

Optional: Meat (one handful—turkey, chicken, or ham are best)

Seasoning (salt, pepper, mustard, Italian dressing, or Parmesan cheese)

### Preparation:

1. Spray skillet.
2. Stir-fry onions for four minutes (at a medium-high temperature).
3. Add chopped broccoli for two minutes; if using meat, add this also.
4. Add can of stewed tomatoes (pour off some excess juice).
5. Break/pour eggs over top; allow to set (harden) for about two minutes.
6. With spatula, swoosh around, maybe flip scoopfuls of it.
7. Add cheese if you insist.
8. Cover and cook on stove top on low until the top sets—or place in the oven on low heat (325°F) for ten to fifteen minutes. When eggs are set all around, you're done.
9. Season (with salt, pepper, mustard, Italian dressing, or Parmesan cheese) to taste.

## Viva Bean Frittata

Spices, corn, and beans make these *huevos* heroic.

### You need:

📎 Skillet and spatula

Cooking spray

Eggs (four, or one eight-ounce carton of egg whites/egg substitute)

Red kidney beans (one can, or black beans)

Green peppers (one bag of frozen; fresh is OK too)

Corn (half a bag, frozen)

Tomatoes (one can stewed or diced)

Small onion (chopped)

Hot sauce, other flavors to taste

Optional: Parmesan cheese

### Preparation:

1. Spray skillet.
2. Stir-fry the onions (on medium high) for four minutes.
3. Add corn, frozen peppers, and stewed tomatoes; stir-fry for four minutes.
4. Add can of beans.
5. Break/pour eggs over top; allow to set (coagulate) for about three minutes.
6. Add cheese if you insist.
7. With spatula, swoosh and flip it around.
8. Cover and cook. When eggs are set all around you're done.
9. Season (with salt, pepper, mustard, hot sauce, or Parmesan cheese) to taste.

Frittatas are good on toast, alongside brown rice, or just by themselves.

### Nuked Eggs

Just as you can do a quick egg on the go in a microwave, you can also do more elaborate dishes there, too—some of them pretty tasty. Just understand, you won't get the crisping effect of frying, and in a round bowl the egg will form this odd mini-soufflé ring. This is due to the outside-in effect of most microwaves; to make sure everything is cooked (to kill off potentially harmful microorganisms, such as *salmonella*), chop up and stir this donut-shaped soufflé midway through the process.

## New Wave Peas 'N Eggs

The sweetness of peas might improve your morning disposition.

### You need:

🖊 Microwavable bowl

Butter or cooking spray

Four eggs or egg-white product

One bag of sweet tender peas (frozen)

Parmesan cheese

Black pepper, salt, other flavors to taste

Optional: small onion, chopped

### Preparation:

1. Coat inside of bowl (with butter or spray).
2. Pour in or beat two eggs (half the egg-white carton), swoosh around inside of bowl.
3. Add bag of frozen peas, liberal amount of Parmesan cheese, seasonings, optional chopped onion.
4. Pour in or add second half of eggs over top of mixture. Mix around.
5. Microwave four minutes; stir, microwave four to six minutes until done.

# NO WHITE CARBS (NWC) PLANS

**N**OTATIONS ARE MADE in some of these recipe for guys attempting the No White Carbs (NWC) plan to lose weight. Basically, this involves the elimination of grain- and potato-based foods, which includes everything from baked goods (bread, muffins, bagels, donuts, cakes, etc.) to cereal to rice to pasta to potatoes (baked, mashed, fried, chips). This is the heart of the high-protein, low-carb Zone diet (and is also a key component of the high-protein, high-fat, low-carb Atkins diet). Ways to do this include substituting vegetables (examples: green leaf vegetables and cooked cabbage) for processed carbohydrates.

Note that the Zone, Atkins, and related approaches dictate a severe restriction on carbohydrates, particularly in the initial phases of the programs. That is neither realistic nor advisable—all the benefits of fruits, vegetables, greens, and whole grains are so well established, benefits such as fiber, flavonoids, phytochemicals, and other components that simply do not exist in animal products. Weight loss or management might be a more gradual process as you follow more balanced structure, but it's an easier-to-maintain "food style" because you are far more likely to continue it into the future.

## SNACKS

There are several convenience foods that serve well as snacks—hard-boiled eggs, protein bars, apples—but during days spent at home it's possible to bump up your snacks to mini-meals. With ready access to a kitchen and groceries, a simple warm snack could be:

Garbanzo beans microwaved with lemon juice and hot sauce (mash with a fork to absorb all the flavors)
Red kidney beans microwaved with frozen corn, flavor at will
Tuna salad mix (cold or microwaved, on bread or alone)
Hard-boiled eggs with Tabasco
Edamame (soybeans in pods, microwaved with vinegar and salt or lemon and black pepper)
Eight-minute cabbage (with a little oil, vinegar, water, salt, and black pepper, microwaved)
Leftovers (cold or microwaved)

What's the difference between a snack and a meal? The threshold between a nibble and dinner is at 200–250 calories.

## LUNCH/DINNER

Meals in this section can be eaten at any time of day.

### Sandwiches

Is there a person who doesn't like sandwiches? As mentioned earlier, they are a pretty perfect mix of nutrition as long as you use the right ingredients. The basic formula:

*Main Stuff:* Tuna, turkey, chicken, ham, sardines, anchovies, lean roast beef, or mashed beans. (How? With a fork, you can mash garbanzo, kidney, or black beans.) Other options include soy-based burgers (there is a broad variety of brands; check Nutrition Facts label for excess fat), canned salmon, canned tuna, canned crab, or cooked, peeled, and deveined frozen shrimp.

*Crunch:* Leafy greens, onions, vegetables (mashed with beans), pickles, nuts, whole-grain bread, green sprouts, carrots, or cucumbers.

*Flavor:* Mustards, horseradish, vinegar, mayo ("light," or in small amounts), ketchup, cheese slices, sauerkraut, ginger, hot sauce, pepperoncini, or hot peppers.

**NWC:** You're not completely out of luck with sandwiches if you're avoiding bread. Just replace two slices of bread with a mashed bean pancake (must be eaten with a fork). Legumes are great food; they're compatible with sandwich ingredients and high in protein and fiber. Some people even use green cabbage or lettuce leaves to make wrap-style sandwiches. Ralph Roberts, proprietor of Vitality Natural Foods in Wilmette, IL, says to discard the outer leaves (which are more acidic) and use the tastier (more alkaline) inner leaves. Don't knock it until you've tried it.

# CHARLIE THE TUNA GIVES PEAS A CHANCE

**A** GUY WITH NO prior cooking skills might do poorly with or be intimidated by seafood. Fish smells bad after three days, and some kinds might kill you—this could mess up a weekend. But tuna is easy—it's what our mothers made us for lunch—so most of us have a warm place in our hearts for the basic tuna sandwich. It's hard to screw up with tuna—even if you do, it's no big loss since the average cost for a big (twelve ounce) can is under $4. You can even just eat it directly from the can (carefully). Mom did all she could to satisfy your undeveloped taste buds, but a guy's job is to take it a step further. Add things that say you've grown up, you are your own man, and, yeah, you like to mix in green stuff. And you don't have to put it on bread, either. Try this:

- Put a can of tuna in a bowl (Main Stuff)
- Put one chopped onion (Flavor and Crunch—any type will do) in the same bowl.
- Put a frozen box of peas (protein, Flavor) in the same bowl.
- Mix in globs of one or several of the following emulsifiers: mustard, ranch dressing, low-fat mayo, Tabasco, or lemon juice (Flavor). Go easy on the quantity; this is not a soup.
- For extra points, add one more thing that's a little weird, like raisins, grapes, or chopped nuts. Tried-and-true celery is always a winner, too—an homage to Mom.

Mix, microwave (option: serve cold but thaw the peas first), and eat from the mixing bowl, or on a tortilla or regular bread (whole grain). Cover leftover portions and store (in an air-tight container) in the refrigerator. Eat leftovers within three days. If you're not sure about the emulsifier and extra-point ingredients, sample these things on the side until you find a combination you like.

## MAKE-AHEAD MEALS

### *Casseroles and one-skillet meals*

Give a man a fish, he eats for a day. Teach a man to fish, he eats for a life-time. When the man learns how to stir-fry, he will figure out how to eat all the damn fish. Tuna is actually a good casserole ingredient. Beans and chicken are, too. All in all, casseroles are a balanced mix of foods that dirty few dishes in the preparation and create excellent convenience when you make enough for several meals at a time.

"Casseroles" might be a misleading word; the casseroles in this book are not swimming in cream of mushroom soup or melted cheese product. These are big-bowl wonders, most often made in a microwave but some-times also stir-fried. Casseroles differ from stir-fried dishes in that they are microwaved; the browning that results from skillet frying will not happen with the microwave method. You could brown an oven-baked casserole, but that would require more time than is likely available in your busy life.

As for serving sizes, with each of these dishes you should eat a protein roughly equivalent to the size of one to two fists. You can eat vegetables to your heart's content. Other tips on portion control: Don't eat while stand-ing up in the kitchen—instead dish up the complete meal onto a plate, sit down, and consider that your dinner. If you are still hungry twenty min-utes after your meal, eat a few more vegetables or move on to an apple, orange, or grapefruit—or maybe a nice peanut butter/yogurt dessert.

Here are some of my favorites:

## Chicken Onion Breath

A basic meal, full of taste, and mind-numbingly simple to make.

### You need:

*Skillet/Chef's pan
  Butter or cooking spray
  Chicken breasts (one to four, frozen)
  Onions (two to three, chopped)
  Balsamic vinegar
  Black pepper, salt, other flavors to taste

Kidney beans (one to two cans)

Green peppers (one bag, frozen)

**Preparation:**

1. Coat inside of skillet (with butter or spray). Set the temperature to medium-high.
2. Stir-fry onions for three minutes. Pour about ⅛ of an inch of vinegar in the skillet.
3. Add chicken breasts (cook for twelve minutes, flip at midpoint).
4. Add green peppers after the chicken has cooked for seven minutes. Reduce heat.
5. Add kidney beans after another three minutes.
6. Scrape the juices out of the pan or deglaze and drip on chicken.

# Pepper Fried Tuna

The rich protein of tuna peppered to give it a good kick.

**You need:**

Skillet/Chef's pan

Butter or cooking spray

Tuna (one or two cans)

Green peppers (one bag, frozen)

Onion (chopped)

Black pepper, salt, other flavors to taste

Balsamic vinegar

Optional: Mushrooms

**Preparation:**

1. Coat skillet (with butter or spray).
2. Stir-fry tuna and onions together for five minutes; add pepper to taste.
3. Add bag of frozen green peppers.
4. Add vinegar (three to five liberal drizzles). Add chopped mushrooms (optional).
5. Stir-fry for another five minutes, with the lid on.
6. Serve; sprinkle with Parmesan cheese and hot sauce.

# Old Wino Chicken

A quick and simple way to make a healthy chicken dish with leftover wine.

### You need:

Microwavable bowl

Chicken breasts (one to two, frozen)

Red wine

Green vegetables (one bag of either broccoli, peas, green peppers, or spinach)

Black pepper, salt, other flavors to taste

### Preparation:

1. Put chicken breasts in bowl; douse with red wine (¼-inch puddle).
2. Sprinkle pepper, salt, and other spices.
3. Microwave four to six minutes. Turn, microwave another two to four minutes.
4. Add green vegetable. Microwave another three to six minutes.
5. Check chicken for doneness (slice one breast in half to see if it's pink on the inside).

# Tuna-on-the-Hoof

Steak sauce is a great way to give tuna a whole new taste. When combined with corn, it's a meal Hoss might have eaten on the Ponderosa ranch.

### You need:

Microwavable bowl

Oil, butter, or cooking spray

Can of tuna

Chopped onion

Steak sauce

Black pepper, salt, garlic, other flavors to taste

Optional: Green vegetables (one bag of either broccoli, peas, green peppers, or spinach)

**Preparation:**
1. Coat inside of bowl (with oil, butter or spray).
2. Empty can of tuna into bowl, with some juices from can. Break up chunks with fork.
3. Add chopped onion and green vegetables (optional).
4. Microwave three to five minutes, more if frozen vegetables are used.
5. Check for doneness.
6. Experiment with small quantities of steak sauce. Use to your taste.

SERVING SUGGESTION: Excellent with steamed corn.

## Plant Protein Palooza

Outta meat? This protein-rich meal is full of surprises when you include the raisins.

**You need:**
Microwavable bowl
Peas (one frozen bag/box)
Kidney beans
Stewed tomatoes (pour off most excess juice)
Oregano, black pepper, salt, other flavors to taste
Brown rice (one cup before cooking)
Raisins (one to two handfuls)
Optional: Small onion, chopped

**Preparation:**
1. Cook rice (according to directions on box); add raisins (large handful) at the end so they don't get too soft.
2. Simultaneously, coat inside of bowl (with oil, butter, or spray)
3. Mix everything together in bowl.
4. Microwave four to eight minutes.
5. Serve large mixture on top of rice/raisin mix.

# Chicken Popeye

Olive oil isn't in this recipe, but Olive Oyl would have eaten it.

### You need:

⚑Microwavable bowl

    Oil, butter, or cooking spray

    Canned chicken (two cans; two breasts of regular chicken can be substituted,
        but then they first need to be cooked)

    One bag of spinach (frozen)

    Kidney or black beans (one to two cans)

    Sun-dried tomatoes, minced (about four small spoonfuls)

    Black pepper, salt, other flavors to taste

    Lemon juice

    Optional: Corn (one bag)

### Preparation:

1. Steam spinach while you work on everything else.
2. Coat inside of bowl (with oil, butter, or spray)
3. Mix canned chicken, beans, two to three doses lemon juice, sun-dried tomatoes, and a little pepper and salt. Microwave four to six minutes.
4. Add a bag of corn, either steamed with the spinach or mixed in with the microwaved chicken (optional).
5. Plate the spinach as a bed; mound everything else on top.

For the spinach-averse, substitute corn or lettuce, or just consider the dish a chicken salad. But give the spinach a shot, at least once.

## Tuna Louisiana

You can turn up the heat as much as you want with extra hot sauce.

### You need:

Saucepan

Brown rice (⅔ cup before cooking)

Tuna (one large can)

Kidney or black beans (one to two cans)

Salsa (twenty-four-ounce jar)

Hot sauce to taste

### Preparation:

1. Cook rice according to directions on box.
2. With three minutes left to cook, add tuna and beans. Finish cooking according to directions.
3. Mix in salsa.
4. Add hot sauce to taste.

*NWC:* The rice is pretty central to this dish, but as long as you use brown or wild rice you are not eating a "white" carb. However, a tuna/beans/salsa mix with some raisins on the side still can be interesting.

## Vampire Be Gone Chicken

Not recommended if you hope to kiss anyone in the next forty-eight hours.

### You need:

Saucepan

Hot chilies (to taste)

Garlic (minced, to taste but start with one large spoonful)

Olive oil

Lemon juice (two dashes)

Chicken breasts (two to four, boneless skinless, frozen)

Green peppers (one bag, frozen)

Stewed tomatoes (one can)

Frozen corn (one bag)

Oregeno

Parmesan Cheese

## Preparation:

1. Coat pan with olive oil; add lemon juice.
2. Stir-fry chilies and garlic at medium-high heat two to three minutes.
3. Add chicken breasts. Braise for six minutes; flip after three minutes. Cook ten to twelve minutes, stirring frequently to avoid burning.
4. Add green peppers, corn, and stewed tomatoes. Cook until corn and peppers are thawed. Check chicken for doneness (slice one breast in half).
5. Eat, perhaps with a little oregano and Parmesan cheese added.
6. Brush teeth and gargle.

# Octopussy Pasta

The high protein of fish in a dish worthy of James Bond.

### You need:

🍳 Saucepan

Seafood medley (frozen bag of seafood: squid, cuttlefish, clams, octopus, mussels, shrimp; 48 grams of protein with only 240 calories in 4 servings, varying somewhat by brand)

Garlic (minced, to taste but start with one large spoonful)

Olive oil

Tomato sauce

Whole-wheat or spinach pasta (prepared according to directions on box)

### Preparation:

1. Coat pan with olive oil.
2. Stir-fry garlic.
3. Add seafood medley. Simmer according to directions on package (about three to five minutes).
4. Add tomato sauce. Simmer for another five to eight minutes.
5. Serve over cooked pasta (or rice).

# DARWIN'S DISH, THE EVOLVING CASSEROLE

**T**HERE IS AN art to using leftovers. Done correctly, a meal can change or grow over several days.

**You need:**

Deep skillet

Chicken breasts (four to five, frozen)

Stewed tomatoes (two cans)

Kidney, garbanzo, or black beans (two cans)

Onions (two, chopped)

**Preparation:**

**1.** *Night One/Creation:* Use your deep skillet to stir-fry some onions, chicken breasts (boneless/skinless), some stewed tomatoes from a can, and a can or two of beans (black, kidney, or garbanzo— whichever appeals at the moment). When the chicken seems sufficiently cooked (if there is no pinkness to the meat), throw a bag of chopped broccoli on top. Eat when broccoli is thawed.

This dish is nice with cold cottage cheese on the side or Parmesan cheese sprinkled on top. Try to eat all the broccoli in this first meal because it tends to turn gray and lose nutrients after cooking.

Assuming you made more than twice as much as needed for a single meal, there will be leftovers to eat later in the week. Store whole skillet in refrigerator, covered.

**2.** *Night Two/Natural Selection:* For the next meal, put the skillet back on the stove and heat (at medium temperature). After a few minutes, throw on a bag of diced peppers, green peas, or some other new vegetable. Cook until thawed. Eat. Finish off the chicken, even if there are beans and tomatoes left in the mix. Try to eat all the green stuff—again, it doesn't hold so well a day after it's cooked. Still have some leftovers? Cover and refrigerate again.

**3.** *Night Three: Modern Times:* For the third meal, heat up what is now beans, tomatoes, and a few errant peas or chopped peppers. Add another can of beans, a bag of frozen corn, and maybe spice it up with hot peppers or hot sauce. Eat. After three meals you should be ready to move on to something different. But notice how each meal was different, and it didn't require much work after the first night.

## Gaga Garbanzoaga

An easy, all-vegetable protein-filled meal in minutes.

### You need:

🖎 Microwavable bowl
    Butter or cooking spray
    Garbanzo beans (two cans)
    Peas (one bag/box, frozen)
    Chopped onion and a little garlic (half a small spoonful)
    Black pepper, salt, other flavors to taste
    Caesar dressing (amount to taste)
    Optional: Parmesan cheese, hot sauce

### Preparation:

1. Coat inside of bowl (with butter or spray).
2. Mix in all ingredients except Parmesan cheese. Go light on the salad dressing—you can always add more later.
3. Microwave four to eight minutes.
4. Add Parmesan cheese, hot sauce (optional).

### Macaroni and Cheese

Let's get something straight here: Mac and cheese violates all the rules. It's heavy on carbs and the "cheese" part is yellow whey dust mixed with butterfat. Just look at the nutrition facts per serving: fourteen grams of protein to ten grams of fat (some brands vary; be wary of brands that do not provide nutritional information after addition of butter and milk). Some ingredients are hydrogenated. It's far from being a nutritional winner when served in its traditional form. But most guys love mac and cheese. So I figure the best we can do is use skim milk and just omit the butter. You will notice that you do not need it anyway if you jazz it up with other things. By making it more interesting you are also diluting the bad with some good. Add any or many of the following:

Chopped broccoli*
Canned beans—especially black or kidney beans
Peas*

Stewed tomatoes
Chopped green peppers*
Hot sauce (or any preferred flavors)
Chopped fresh onions
Tuna
Chicken (pre-cooked, chopped to bite-sized pieces)
Apple slices
Lime juice

*If using the frozen version, either steam separately or toss in with
boiling macaroni in last two minutes.

**NWC:** Skip this; you shouldn't be eating macaroni.

### Soups, Chilis, and Stews

Sure, there are lots of commercially prepared soups out there, with all the
chopping and mixing done for you. But most of them taste terrible, and
despite some of their brand names, none of them are nearly as chunky as
what you can make on your own.

These soups are essentially broth-based, not creamy (creamy soups are
almost always higher in fat). Essential components are water,
broth/stock, vegetables, spices, and usually (but not always) a meat. Be
bold and experiment—discover how easily different flavors, crunchy
foods, and main ingredients can mix together.

## Basic Soup

Hot soup on a cold day—as easy to eat as it is to make.

### You need:

Large kettle (stockpot)

Soup stock (two cans, either beef or chicken)

Vegetables (two bags frozen, your choice)

Beans (One to two cans, your choice)

Meat (bite-sized chunks of chicken, pre-cooked; or beef, cooked in the soup
broth)

Black pepper, salt, other flavors to taste

Optional: Celery (chopped), stewed tomatoes

**Preparation:**

1. Pour soup stock into large kettle; add spices of choice. Bring to a boil on high, then reduce to medium heat.
2. If cooking beef, add to stock for five to ten minutes.
3. Add bag of frozen vegetables and beans; if using pre-cooked chicken, add with vegetables.
4. Simmer until vegetables are thawed, about three to five minutes.

*To pre-cook chicken:*

Put one-to-three frozen chicken breasts in a microwavable bowl. Douse with vinegar (¼-inch puddle), cover with paper towel, and microwave, approximately four minutes per breast (turn at midpoint). When done, slice into bite-sized chunks.

## Tomato Fiesta Soup

Arriba! Arriba! Fast and fiery.

**You need:**
🔖 Large kettle (stockpot)
Stewed tomatoes (two to three cans)
Water (one to two cans)
Green peppers (one to two bags frozen, chopped)
Beans (two cans, garbanzo or others)
Salsa (or spicy tomato sauce, with a chopped onion and hot sauce added)
Chilies, black pepper, salt, other flavors to taste
Optional: Celery (chopped)

**Preparation:**

1. Pour stewed tomatoes and water into stockpot. Bring to a boil on high, then reduce to medium heat.
2. Add green peppers, beans, chilies (chopped), and other seasonings.
3. Simmer and stir until vegetables are thawed, about three to five minutes.

# BORN-AGAIN DOGGIE BAG

**I**T LOOKS LIKE you were thinking with your beer brain again. So juicy, tasty, and big, that curved edge calling your name—you woke up with a little shame and regret, and now you have remnants of your obsession. You ate about three-quarters of that pizza last night. What should you do with the leftovers?

Pizza has some great, healthful components—tomatoes, onions, olive oil—but in one-slice-per-day portions. Try to spread the slices out over two or three days with the sin-dilution method previously discussed for macaroni and cheese. Here are a few ideas:

■ Create a protein-rich mash, such as with tuna or a garbanzo/spices mix. Spread the mash on a leftover pizza slice.

■ Chop the pizza leftovers into bite-sized pieces, then sprinkle those over a mixed green salad along with sliced tomatoes and one or two cans of beans (kidney, garbanzo, black).

■ Make a pizza chicken sandwich, with microwaved chicken breasts placed between two slices. This gets messy, so don't think you can eat it in the living room without a big plate.

But what about other kinds of leftovers? What do you do with doggie-bag meat, pasta, or rice? From your own kitchen, almost everything in this book (except oatmeal) can be refrigerated for later consumption. Things brought home from a restaurant should be re-served with greens and other vegetables. A creamy pasta dish such as an alfredo is a bit more challenging: Try the mac-and-cheese tactics if you insist on eating all those simple carbs.

## Red Chicken Soup

Tangy tomatoes and balsamic chicken make for one savory soup.

### You need:

✎ Saucepan–large kettle (stockpot) if you make a larger quantity
    Chicken stock (chicken bouillon cubes can be substituted for stock, but will
        tend to make the soup saltier)
    Stewed tomatoes (one can)
    Beans (one can, garbanzo or other types)
    Cooked chicken (two breasts, microwaved with balsamic vinegar)
    Black pepper, salt, oregano
    Optional: Celery (chopped)

### Preparation:

1. Pour soup stock into saucepan or stockpot; add spices. Bring to a boil on high, then reduce to medium heat.
2. Simultaneously microwave chicken in balsamic vinegar (six to ten minutes, turn at midpoint).
3. Add stewed tomatoes and beans; simmer on medium-low heat.
4. Add chicken (chopped into bite-sized pieces) and juices from microwaved bowl.
5. Serve with oyster crackers and Parmesan cheese.

See chapter 13 for large-kettle recipes good enough for company or to be consumed by one self-respecting guy over several days.

### *Full Meals*

Ah, picture it. After an invigorating, productive workday and a surprisingly rigorous workout at the gym, you arrive home to wonderful smells wafting from the kitchen, announcing a meal timed for your arrival.

Dream on. You ain't Ward Cleaver. No one's cooking for you. These are recipes for the guy who yearns for a fresh meal, where the meat stands on its own with other things on the side. Note that for most meat dishes, the George Foreman-style clamshell grill cooks red meat, chicken, and fish quickly. But a skillet accommodates cooking with onions and other flavors. All recipes here are written for the traditional skillet.

# Basic Salmon

Nutritious, tasty, and relatively easy to make—a guy's perfect dinner.

### You need:

🍴 Skillet

    Salmon fillets or steaks*

    Olive oil (another option is to rub the raw fish on the pan; its natural fat can
       do the trick)

    Onion (chopped)

    Salt, pepper, and spices to taste (garlic if you like)

    Fresh lime or lime juice

### Preparation:

1. Chop onion.
2. Oil skillet (just enough to coat the bottom); set to medium heat.
3. Stir-fry onion and spices in pan for two to four minutes.
4. Sprinkle salt and pepper over salmon fillets.
5. Cook salmon in skillet (covered with lid) for two minutes on each side.
6. Squeeze lime over cooked salmon.

*Four ounces of fish has between twenty and thirty-two grams of protein, depending on the type. Canned, frozen, and fresh fish have approximately the same nutritional makeup.

SUGGESTED SIDE DISH: Steamed vegetables (broccoli, peas, cauliflower, green beans, asparagus). Drippings from the pan can be used to flavor a side dish. Pour a wineglass full of wine (red or white) in with the drippings; lower heat and simmer for an interesting mix of flavor. This is called deglazing.

## Basic Chicken

So easy and quick, you can make and eat this while talking on the phone.

### You need:

🖎 Skillet

Olive oil

Chicken breasts (two frozen, boneless/skinless)

Salt, pepper, and spices to taste

Optional: Onion (chopped) and/or garlic

### Preparation:

1. Chop onion (optional).
2. Oil skillet (just enough to coat the bottom); set to medium heat.
3. Put onion and spices in pan; cook for one to three minutes.
4. Place chicken breasts in skillet; braise for two minutes on each side (raise to high heat), then cook on medium until done (approximately ten minutes total).

SUGGESTED SIDE DISH: Steamed vegetables (broccoli, peas, cauliflower, green beans, asparagus).

## Basic Skillet-Fried Steaks

Delicious, fast, and satisfying.

### You need:

🖎 Skillet

Lean cut of meat: top sirloin, top loin, T-bone, or tenderloin

Salt, pepper, and spices to taste (garlic if you like)

Optional: Butter (one to two pats)

### Preparation:

1. Rub meat around surface of pan; or use one to two pats of butter (optional).

2. Heat skillet on medium.
3. Sear* each side of steak in pan for two to three minutes (raise heat to high).
4. Reduce heat to medium. Sprinkle with salt and pepper to taste.
5. Cook meat (covered) to preferred doneness.

*Searing is a short, hot exposure to the outside of a piece of meat that effectively seals in its natural juices. Be sure to do both sides.

SUGGESTED SIDE DISH: Steamed vegetables (broccoli, peas, cauliflower, green beans, asparagus).

# HOW LONG SHOULD I COOK A STEAK?

**RARE:** eight to twelve minutes
**MEDIUM:** thirteen to sixteen minutes
**WELL DONE:** twenty minutes

## Side Dishes

Animal protein needs the balance of plant foods, of course. But you don't have to eat just one vegetable—you can jazz them up by making different combinations:

Corn and sauerkraut
Corn and black beans
Broccoli and diced chili peppers
Broccoli and sun-dried tomatoes
Cauliflower with lemon and Parmesan cheese
Peas and garbanzo beans
Peas and sauerkraut
Peas and one or two types of beans
Green beans mixed with other types of beans
Cooked brown rice mixed with carrots and raisins
Cooked brown rice with virtually any vegetable
Spinach and beans
Spinach and corn
Spinach and light mayonnaise

# AVOIDING LEFTOVER SICKNESS

**A**CCORDING TO AN urban legend, more people die each year from mayonnaise gone bad than from shark attacks. From a Kraft Foods Web site, here's a list of smart leftover-management practices to help you (and dinner guests) avoid driving the porcelain bus.

- Refrigerate or freeze leftovers within two hours.
- Cool leftovers quickly. Before refrigerating or freezing, slice large cuts of meat and store in serving-size packets; use small containers to store stews and chilis.
- Label leftovers with the current date. Eat or freeze within three to four days.
- Check the refrigerator once a week and discard old leftovers. When in doubt, throw it out.
- Reheat leftovers until piping hot all the way through.

When re-serving, kill residual microorganisms with these techniques:

- Cover food with a vented covering.
- Rotate food halfway through cooking time.
- Stir food halfway through cooking time (even if microwave has a turntable).
- Stir food again after cooking is completed.
- Allow food to stand for five minutes after cooking.
- Never reheat leftovers in a slow cooker. The gradual heating promotes bacterial growth.

Additionally, store food in the correct-size containers. Too much air will encourage the growth of bacteria. If the container is too small, the cover might not fit tightly, and this can also cause contamination.

Most leftovers taste great and most people survive intact. Treat them right and you'll have little to worry about.

### Desserts

If you eat smart all day long, will a small bowl of ice cream at night blow it? In the strictest sense, no. Your body metabolizes food in a sum-total fashion, so the nutritional pluses balance against the minuses. If ice cream is a major love of your life, then have at it. Just be cognizant of the portion size—one cup per evening won't kill you, but note also that there are *four* cups in those little pint packages.

Then consider how a no-fat, no-sugar-added yogurt would allow you a bit more bulk and add rather than subtract from overall nutrition. Or give moderation a shot. Maybe instead of ice cream five nights a week, try a schedule that has you eating fruit two nights a week, or at least fruit and a half-portion of ice cream. If you discover you can manage a change in routine—and you like the math of more nutrients, fewer calories, and fewer fat grams—we have a few ideas that you might try:

### Mostly Fruit Desserts

You can get part of your nine-a-day fruits and vegetables in a dessert if you're smart. Following are some easy, two-minute wonders:

Apple slices, sprinkled with sweetener and cinnamon, then
    microwaved for about a minute
Orange slices, drizzled with melted peanut butter
Grapefruit sections with walnuts and brown sugar
Bananas with melted peanut butter and strawberries

### Low-Fat Yogurt and Cottage Cheese

Fat replacement in dairy products—where all-protein non-fat whey mimics the creaminess of traditional butterfat—makes low-fat dessert pretty easy. My favorites:

⊃ *Yogurt/Peanut Butter Pull:* The dessert you eat when no one else is looking. Start with a large spoonful of peanut butter, and dip into a tub of fat-free yogurt (plain, vanilla, or flavored). Insert glob in mouth and, using teeth and lips, gently pull off the layer of yogurt and just a bit of the peanut butter. Return spoonful of (diminishing) peanut butter into yogurt and repeat the process until peanut butter is gone (five to eight pulls).

⊃ *Yogurt/Applesauce Mix:* Combine equal quantities of yogurt and applesauce on a small plate. Add cinnamon and raisins.

⊃ *Cottage Cheese and Fruit:* Raisins, apple slices, bananas, strawberries, and anything else combined with fat-free cottage cheese makes a fruit/protein dessert that is so darn wholesome, you could eat it for breakfast. Add sweetener to taste.

⊃ *Protein Monkey*: Smashed banana, protein powder, and yogurt, mixed to a smooth, delicious consistency. This can be frozen for eating later if you don't mind a little ice crystallization.

## WHAT TO DO WHEN MEALS GO WRONG?

EVEN THE BEST COOKS make mistakes, and if you're experimenting you'll probably make a few yourself. Here are some tips for picking up the pieces when your meal lets you down.

1.  Assess the mistake: Was it poor-quality ingredients? Bad combinations? Was something missing? Was the food overcooked or undercooked? This is an analytical task the engineers should find invigorating.
2.  Salvage it—add something (or take something out?). Too much salt? Add other non-salty things to dilute the problem. Bland taste? Add salt, pepper, or other herbs and spices—it could be a good opportunity to experiment. Too hot (spicy)? Add crackers or other grainy foods (breads, rice, or pasta) to neutralize it.
3.  Next time, make components separately, then mix samples together, one by one, to find the taste that works.

After all, if you don't make meals you're going to want again, you'll be headed back to Burgerville pretty fast.

# 12

# a guy's gotta cook for a date

## Just making the effort can win her heart

**Ask five women** the following question: Is it especially romantic when a guy cooks for you? Chances are that four if not all five will say yes. The theory that food = love is hardly new. In a simpler time, it was a given that the way to a man's heart was through his stomach. Feminism challenged all that, of course, which opens the opportunity for us to turn the tables: The way to a woman's heart is through *her* stomach.

Well, maybe not. Women have a thing about their stomachs. Guys, too. So I'll rephrase it: "The road to love is paved with an appetizer, a salad, and a good, nutritious entrée, followed by a nice, light dessert. Wine is optional but encouraged." What it lacks in poetry it makes up for in simple instruction. There is actual data culled from a little survey I did while writing this book to support the idea. I asked a few questions of women at farmers' markets in Chicago and New York City because I guessed they would have discerning interests in food. Thirty-seven women and one gay man, appearing to be between the ages of twenty-something and fifty-something, answered these questions: How often do you shop at a farmers' market? What is your primary purpose for being here? Do you see men you find attractive here? And does the fact that a guy shops for food at a farmers' market enhance his attractiveness? A fifth question was open-ended, allowing them to elaborate on what it is that makes a man appealing when shopping for fresh fruits and vegetables.

The responses in both cities were similar and resolute.

⊃ This is a regular crowd. Three-quarters (76 percent) indicated they were there weekly; another 13 percent were there about once a month. So if someone catches your eye but you're feeling shy, there's a good chance she'll be back next week.

⊃ The primary purpose for being there was "fresh food" (68 percent) followed by "food and social, to mix with friends and neighbors" (18 percent).

⊃ Their eyes are on more than the tomatoes. About two-thirds (63 percent) reported that they do spot a looker here and there. A quarter (24 percent) said that they never notice such things or are not looking (marital status was not a screen, therefore respondents may be off the market and completely enamored with their partners, or bitter beyond hope). The bottom line is that there's a lot more going on behind their sunglasses than you might at first guess.

⊃ When asked, "Does the fact that a guy shops for food at a farmers' market enhance his attractiveness?", a full *87 percent* said yes. This seems to directly relate to the famous Woody Allen axiom that 85 percent of life is a matter of just showing up.

The reasons given for the "yes" response in the fourth question told a bigger story. Here are some comments to the final, open-ended question:

"I'm interested in food, and if a guy is interested in food, we have a shared interest."

"Men who cook are sexy."

"He takes care of himself; he puts an effort into it. He might also be interested in the environment."

"He's adventurous, knows what's going on in the city, and is health-conscious."

"He is interested in healthy foods and in supporting local farmers."

"An interest in food shows he has depth—and, hopefully, he can cook!"

"It's great when someone cooks for you, and someone who shops here would cook."

"People who shop here care about good food and care about their bodies."

"Anyone who shops for fresh food is attractive and has some knowledge of what he's doing."

"Anyone interested in food is interested in life. He likes the outdoors and has an appealing personality."

"Guys here take the time to do this sort of thing versus the lazy guys at home."

"He might know something about food, not always eating fast food. Food is a big thing for me!"

"This shows a guy is thoughtful and mature, thinking of more than beer. But does it mean he's looking to pick up a girl [if he comes to the farmers' market]?"

"Guys here are out doing everyday fun things in a natural environment."

"I wish there were more men here!"

There are some key things a guy can take away from this. First, farmers' markets are a gold mine of women who are predisposed to noticing guys (note that the gender mix at these Saturday morning markets seems to be about 70/30, female/male). And just sniffing a few cantaloupes might be all you have to do. Also, it's casual weekend dress, so a pair of jeans, a sweatshirt, and a baseball cap pretty much covers you. Shaving is optional. (Beer-brand and Taco Bell T-shirts are not advised.) A guy like you would be interesting, approachable, and ripe for casual conversation, which might go as follows:

YOU: "I see you got the grapes. Are they good this week?"
HER: "Oh, yes."
YOU: "Boy, it's good to get them when they're in season. And I like helping the local farmers."

YOU: "Hello. How are those blueberries?"
HER: "Pretty good. Here, try one."
YOU: "This must be the peak week. They're sweet and juicy—and I like the antioxidants. Sure beats ice cream, chips, or beer. Hey, try this basil . . . ."

YOU: "Where did you get your apple cider?"
HER: "Uh, at that stand over there. They have samples."
YOU: "Cool. Cider always reminds me of my grandmother's apple trees back upstate, which we grew organically. Maybe it's because I spent so much time there working on the farm as a kid that now I'm just not the kind of guy who sits around on a couch."

HER: "Are those beefsteak tomatoes? Where did you get them?"
YOU: "I'm not sure what kind they are. They're from that stand right over there."
HER: "They look like beefsteak. Those are great on barbecued hamburgers."
YOU: "I'll have to try that. You probably know how to grill vegetables."

And so on. Even hammy lines like these can be charming when she knows you eat smart simply because you are at this market.

Almost anywhere you live, chances are there is a farmers' market not too far away—it is a food-retailing phenomenon on the rise. The number of farmers' markets in the United States has increased by 79 percent since 1994, reports the U.S. Department of Agriculture, to more than 3,100 such markets in all 50 states. While largely restricted to the harvest periods (midsummer through the first frost or when the crops are done), about three million Americans shop at one each week during the season.

Note that the idea of shopping at a farmers' market is consistent with your usual habit of working with long-shelf-life foods. There's nothing wrong with truly fresh foods; you simply have to eat them within a few days (the reason most market shoppers return week after week). Farmers' market produce (and organic or range-raised meats, sold at some markets) is a great supplement to the frozen and canned goods you already have in stock—for a few days, at least, you can savor the tastes and textures not generally available in a supermarket. You are getting food picked within the past day or two when buying direct from local farmers. And you might even meet a nice, healthy girl while you're at it.

## THE ELEMENTS OF DINNER-DATE COOKING

YOUR SMART EATING STRUCTURE will work exceptionally well when making dinner for a date. Even if they don't in fact eat smart on their own, most women want everyone else to believe they eat like delicate hummingbirds (birds that in fact consume up to three times their body weight every day). So allow them to keep that perception intact by serving healthy foods—chances are you'll have plenty of leftovers for later.

Many of the recipes included in chapters 11 and 13 are fine for date food, but the dishes found in this chapter are more appropriate for serving to others, particularly in a romantic situation. New ideas presented here are going to expand your repertoire of cooking skills.

The date-night dinner will also require a little more time and possibly a few additional grocery items. Fresh greens are an easy, no-lose proposition— and not much work if you buy the pre-chopped, -washed, and -mixed kind. Fresh herbs (cilantro, basil, rosemary) may seem like a small thing to you but to the supertaster (women tend to have more sensitive taste buds) they can be a rock-my-world experience. By now, you know where the grocery store is, so study your intended recipes a day or two in advance to see what new items you'll need.

There are five things you need to consider in preparing for a dinner date. They are:

1. Mood and atmosphere
2. Make-ahead food (salad, dressings, side dishes, etc.)
3. Main dish (to be cooked fresh)

4. Beverage
5. Dessert

The impression you want to convey in all of this is ease, control, a sense of pleasure, and healthiness, and yet that this dinner is not something you have done for many other people before. Few people expect men to have cooking skills. It's a misconception, actually sexist, but it works in your favor. The pressure's off; the mere fact you are making the effort gives you points. A little overcooking or under-salting will not kill the evening—in fact, a small goof here and there handled correctly can be endearing. Enjoy the whole process—preparation, eating, and post-meal—because an at-home dinner date is as much about the journey as the destination, much like many things in life and gastronomy.

## 1. MOOD AND ATMOSPHERE

There is no "rules" book for men looking to land a trophy partner, and can we all just be a little thankful for that? After all, the business of dating and romance should have a certain "just be you" quality. But it's a realm of best impressions and behaviors, so there are some things you should attend to prior to setting up an at-home romance:

***Clean floors, kitchen, bathroom—and the air:*** This includes porcelain surfaces; they should be free of anything other than the porcelain. Elsewhere around the house, scraps of meals past, lint from laundry in the carpet, and all pet hairs (as well as hairs of your last date) need to go. Commercial carpet-spot removers work very well and take mere seconds to apply. As for air quality, the most likely pitfalls are as follows: bad kitchen odors (a full garbage can, dirty sink drains, rotten fruit or vegetables, or lingering aromas from fish or garlic made in the three days prior to the date night), bad pet odors, and bad bathroom odors. In the kitchen, a good cleaning with lemon-scented products can do wonders fast. The latter two problems should be addressed with open windows an hour or two before your date arrives, emptying of cat boxes, use of carpet and upholstery sprays, and a slow-burning scented candle in the bathroom, lit before your guest arrives.

***Tidy up:*** Put books onto bookshelves, magazines in neat stacks, and keep newspapers and junk mail hidden away or sent to recycling. Put clothes in the hamper, and close closet doors. Your home does not need to be sterile—in fact, a little character should show through—but don't make your guest trip over anything out of place.

***Adjust lighting:*** Few people like bright, fluorescent lights. Women in particular have an issue about this. Something about the light of fluorescent bulbs can make even Brandi Chastain appear wan. Bright incandescent overhead lights can be equally disconcerting, as they bring out complexion flaws, real or perceived; dim, indirect lights are much more forgiving. If your kitchen and dining room have only the former, move a floor or desk lamp in for softer dinner lighting. Try lots of candles, which are a cheap and easy trick—just keep it to less than ten, lest you appear to be following a Caribbean-based religion (acceptable, of course, if indeed you do).

***Turn on music:*** Taste in music is much like taste in food—much of it is personal. Angry rap is generally not a good idea for a romantic dinner; the same can be said of 70s acid rock and vintage disco. Or maybe not. Playing Enya might be asking too much of you, but perhaps you should look at it as a means to an end. Mozart is more appropriate for brunch. Tenors singing opera in their incessantly dramatic way might get you some truck. If your date offers to bring anything, suggest she bring a few CDs of her choosing.

***Set the table:*** No one expects you to have matching tableware, since you probably have not yet gone through the whole wedding shower bonanza. If you *have* and are single again, it would surprise no one if you chose the dog over stemware in the settlement. You need the basics: dinner plates, flatware (knives, forks, and spoons), salad/dessert plates (or bowls), drinking glasses, and wineglasses. Even if they are not part of a set, at least try to have same elements match up (same wineglasses, same plates, same forks, etc.).

Then there's the question about foofy accessories on the table. First, they need not be foofy. A tablecloth might not even be necessary. Rustic is "in." Under some circumstances a beach towel might serve as a good tablecloth. Or the unprinted side (inside) of flattened brown grocery bags. It's safest to go with just the naked table surface. As for the decoration, try any of the following:

⊃ A grouping of thick, beer can–width candles—at least three but not occupying more than about 10 percent of the table surface.

You still need room for the food. It's arty if the candles are of different heights. Or use long-burning tall candles; if you lack candleholders, beer bottles (with the labels removed) might do the trick. Votives, the stubby long-burning candles, can be purchased in bulk; put five or six on a plate and call it a day.

⊃ A bowl filled with colorful things from nature. Fruit works, of course, as do fallen leaves and cut flowers (enough blooms to fill the bowl). Heck, try fruit and leaves, or fruit and flowers, or leaves and flowers. Dandelions could earn you points for cuteness. Even live goldfish. Lately, an actual section of sod, growing grass, seems to be in vogue, although to me it seems a lot like a Chia Pet. Don't get a Chia Pet.

⊃ Plants you can eat. Many grocery stores carry rosemary, thyme, and sage plants—herbs you can snip from the plant and put directly on your food. I have a rosemary plant that I bought two years ago; with minimal care it continues to live and in fact thrive because I trim a few twigs now and then to flavor chicken. Cultivating your own herbs puts you in a league of your own.

The objective in setting the mood is to evoke a style that is consistent with your personality. Cool understatement is probably your best bet, but that all depends. If you can pull off kitsch and it gets you action, go with it.

## 2. MAKE-AHEAD FOOD

The message you want to impart is that this dinner was a labor of love, yet somehow effortless. You want your focus to be on your date instead of the onions. And you don't want to have a layer of sweat on your face. A solution is to make some stuff ahead of time. The success of most meals depends on the quality of the meat or other "Main Stuff"—where juiciness, tenderness, flavor, and temperature really count—and therefore the make-ahead portion should be appetizers, green salad, and side dishes. Here's a list of what you can include:

### Appetizers
⊃ Baby carrots and green pepper slices, served with hummus dip (commercially prepared).

⊃ Apple or pear slices with a yogurt dip or cheddar cheese (get the brick cheese, not wrapped slices).

⊃ Shrimp, served on ice to give the impression of hygiene and microbiological control; serve cocktail sauce alongside, in a small bowl or plain coffee cup. Girls love shrimp because it's a high-protein, low-fat treat (but, an anomaly in nature, it is high in cholesterol).

### Green Salad or Soup

It is hard to go wrong with green salad, as long as you stay away from iceberg lettuce (nutritionally speaking, iceberg is little more than water and a tiny bit of fiber; other types of greens carry more nutrients and taste—the darker in color the better). Salad clearly communicates that you think about smart nutrition. Just wash it and break it up by hand into fork-ready pieces. Salad dressings can include prepared commercial types or oil/vinegar/spice mixes you make yourself (it's very easy to do; see recipes on page 194).

Soup, such as chicken minestrone, would be a handy alternative under several circumstances; for example, when you don't have time to get the fresh ingredients required for a salad. In colder-weather months, soup is a warm-the-heart kind of dish. Served with whole-grain bread, it's a meal (for extra points, warm the bread in the oven or toaster).

### Side Dishes

Keeping within the *A Guy's Gotta Eat* structure, your side dishes should include Flavor and Crunch. Clearly, vegetables and maybe a whole-grain component are in order. But be sure the side dish contains almost none of the ingredients used in the main dish (e.g., don't serve chicken soup with a chicken main dish; don't flavor a side dish with lemon juice when the main dish also uses lemon or lime). Therefore, you should decide what your main dish will be first, then work backward from there. The following side dishes are suggested, with recipes at the end of this chapter:

Multi-Bean Salad
Wild Rice and Broccoli
Maize Craze
Teutonic Corn

Pea Garbanzo Fiesta
Couscous on the Loose
Grilled Vegetables
Tomato Potato
Pasta (Whole Wheat or Spinach)

## 3. MAIN DISH (TO BE COOKED FRESH)

Because you'll be making this in the middle of your date, the dish should be fairly simple to prepare and not too time-consuming. Save the soufflé or lamb flambé for when you have hired help; most of this is Main Stuff that involves less than fifteen minutes of heat and no more than a handful of ingredients. Recipes begin on page 205.

## 4. BEVERAGE

The question of what to drink is complicated. Your acuity at avoiding a date faux pas can be increased by asking the following questions:

⊃ Is your date a recovering alcoholic (or teetotaler)? If either, think about grape juice, herbal tea, filtered, sparkling, or bottled water.

⊃ Have you been with your date socially before and observed her drink of preference? A simple drink (gin and tonic, scotch and soda) might be replicated at home; you are not expected to create anything involving umbrellas.

⊃ What about wine? Do you have a *clue*? If so, go with what you know; the advice given here may be too basic for you. If not, here are some guidelines to follow: nothing in a box, and you would do well to avoid jug wines as well. Women seem to like white wines more than most men do, but that's a broad generalization with many exceptions. The drier (less sweet) reds seem to go well with most meals: these include Merlot, Pinot Noir, Shiraz, and Cabernet Sauvignon varieties. Spend a minimum of $8 per bottle; if you don't know much about what you are serving, don't try to fake it. The only thing worse than a wine snob is a fake oenophile. Should your date ask something like, "Is this Chilean?" you should pause quizzically, then say, "I dunno. I asked the guy at the store for something that goes good with [name of main dish]." This not only lets you off the hook from groping your way through a wine conversation; it shows that you were thinking about this meal a day or two in advance. Additionally, if your date knows wine and was working toward criticizing the choice (rude, but seemingly a habit of wine-knowledgeable types), only the liquor-store clerk is to blame.

⊃ Of course, always serve water at the dinner table. I have a theory that it is smarter to drink water after dinner (I think your mouth's saliva should continue to be stimulated by food tastes, even after you've swallowed, to aid digestion), but social convention requires that you give your guests the option of drinking water with dinner.

## 5. DESSERT

If your guest brings a cake or ice cream, go ahead and serve it. But remembering how high-sugar foods can wreck a mood, dessert can be a critical part of the meal: Make it sweet without sending your date into a post-dinner blood-sugar coma. Also note that each dish is very simple and can be made with ingredients you already have on hand. Suggestions begin on page 210.

Nutritious eating may not guarantee you some action, but following a few simple, tactical maneuvers should increase your odds.

## DATE-NIGHT RECIPES FOR SUCCESS

IF YOU'VE BEEN WORKING with the guidelines and recipes laid down in chapter 11, these dishes are just a few steps up in methods and ingredients. To avert a panicked, last-minute dash to the grocery store, ingredients that were not specified in chapter 9 are printed here in **boldfaced type**.

## MAKE-AHEAD FOOD: Salad, Dressings, and Soup

### Green Salad

THE FIRST FEW TIMES you prepare this salad, go with pre-mixed greens, sometimes called "**mesclun**." Other mixed greens come bagged, including fresh spinach. The mix is interesting to the eye as well as the palate. Try to purchase this, whether sold in bulk or pre-bagged, and other fresh ingredients the day that you'll serve them—greens wilt (and lose nutrients) rapidly with time. Steps to help you serve it well:

- ⊃ Wash and rinse, using your colander or steam insert to drain.
- ⊃ Add a few things to give it more texture and flavor; try **fresh tomatoes**, garbanzo or kidney beans, chopped onions, or corn (add frozen; it will thaw within twenty minutes).
- ⊃ Store with a cover of wet paper towels in refrigerator until ready to serve.
- ⊃ Serve with **tongs** or **salad-service utensils**.
- ⊃ Got leftovers? Put wet paper towels over greens (store leftover dressing separately); cover with plastic wrap. If there are fresh tomatoes in the mix, it helps to remove them (acidity of tomatoes causes quicker degeneration of the greens).

## Salad Dressing

### *Oil/Vinegar/Spice Mixes (Optional: Oil/Lemon Juice/Spice Mix)*

A simple vinaigrette dressing takes about twenty-three seconds to make, using olive oil, vinegar (balsamic or other), and spices (any chopped herbs, salt, pepper, and a smidgen of mustard or some commercially prepared dried-spice packets). Or substitute lemon juice for vinegar, an advisable alternative if your main dish has a strong vinegary taste. Steps:

1. In a tall jar or glass (e.g., a recycled tomato sauce jar), put equal parts oil and vinegar (start with a half-shot glass or two dashes of each).
2. Add spices, dried or fresh.
3. Swoosh in glass in a rotating motion, aided by a spoon.
4. You and your date should pour or spoon on to the greens just as you are ready to eat.

## Citrus Vinaigrette*

Orange, lime, and mustard give this dressing a strong and complex taste, something to savor as you eat your salad.

### You need:
 Large jar

    Orange juice (half a coffee cup full)

    Lime juice (three big spoonfuls)

    Olive oil (two big spoonfuls)

    Mustard (**Dijon-style**, one big spoonful)

### Preparation:
1. Mix all ingredients in jar.
2. Stir vigorously, then pour on individual salads.

*Recipe used with permission from the Bean Education & Awareness Network; recommended for use with a tuna-bean salad.

## Love Soups
THESE CAN BE MADE ahead and reheated, or served as the main meal.

## Nona Bravo's Chicken Minestrone

She came to America at the age of twelve with little more than the dreams in her heart and some recipes in her satchel. Today, Nona's grandson Eddie fiercely maintains the true art of minestrone (note that "minestrone" means "big soup" in Italian, but often also means "clean up what's left over in the kitchen"). This soup can be served before dinner in place of a salad or alone, as a nice, casual meal (cue the Pavarotti CD).

### You need:
Saucepan

Chicken (two to four breasts, pre-cooked in skillet with vinegar–the chicken can be microwaved, but Eddie says Nona would throw a Neapolitan fit at the idea) cut into bite-sized pieces.

Chicken broth (two cans)

Stewed tomatoes (one can)

**Beans** (one to two cans **navy** or kidney beans)

Salt, pepper, oregano, and other "Italian seasonings" to taste

Pasta that can cook in six to ten minutes (about 1½ coffee cups full, read directions on side of box; it's important to use small pasta, such as **ditalini** or **elbow**)

Vegetables (frozen, two to three bags broccoli, cauliflower, or green beans cut into bite-sized pieces)

Optional: Parmesan cheese, **cornstarch** (⅓ coffee cup full)

### Preparation:

1. Pour chicken broth, tomatoes, beans, and seasonings into pan.
2. Heat on high until it boils.
3. Add vegetables and pasta to mix. Cook about eight to ten minutes.
4. When pasta is cooked, add chicken.
5. Add cornstarch to thicken as needed (optional).
6. Sprinkle with Parmesan cheese (optional).

## Sweet Potato Chicken Soup

Another warm-the-heart favorite, you can make it spicy or mild— check to see if your date likes things mild, medium, or hot.

### You need:

Deep skillet

Olive oil (one dash)

Chicken (two to four breasts, frozen)

Onion (one, chopped)

Chicken broth (one can, plus one to two cans water)

Sweet potatoes (two large, cut to bite-size cubes)

Stewed tomatoes (one can)

Salt, pepper, and crushed red peppers to taste (mild, medium, or hot)

Optional: Parmesan cheese, chopped celery, chopped cilantro

**Preparation:**

1. Chop onion and stir-fry in olive oil and spices for two to five minutes on medium-high heat.
2. Pour chicken broth and water into skillet and add frozen chicken breasts. Heat on medium-high until it boils.
3. Chop onions and cut sweet potatoes into cubes (leave skin on but scrub and remove roots and blemishes). Add to skillet.
4. Add chopped celery (optional).
5. Cook until chicken is done; test by cutting through the middle of one breast. Use flat end of a spatula to chop chicken into bite-sized pieces.
6. Add chopped cilantro as you serve the soup (optional).

Note: Cooked chicken in soups does not need to be uniformly chopped into neat little cubes. Haphazard bite-sized pieces enhance the home-made quality.

## Side Dishes

MOST OF THESE can be prepared in bulk and eaten all week.

## Multi-Bean Salad

A '50s favorite re-made for today—packed with protein, fiber, and complex carbohydrates, the smart date will recognize your intelligence when you serve this wholesome dish.

**You need:**

Vegetable steamer/saucepan

Olive oil (one shot glass full)

Red wine vinegar (two shot glasses full)

Green beans (one bag)*

**Yellow beans** (TIP: these look just like green beans, only yellow; two handfuls, generally sold fresh or in cans)*

Red kidney beans (one can)

Green pepper (one bag chopped)

Red onion (chopped)

Salt, pepper, seasonings to taste (recommended: **fresh cilantro**, chopped)

Optional: **sugar** (¾ coffee cup full).

*If green and/or yellow beans are not available, substitute garbanzo and black beans.

### Preparation:
1. Steam-cook beans (green and yellow).
2. Combine all ingredients in a large bowl; mix (if sugar is used, make sure it is dissolved and evenly distributed).
3. Refrigerate; can be made a day in advance. Serve cold.

# CHOPPING HERBS

**I** USED TO SPEND way too much time separating leaves from stalks on cilantro and other fresh herbs until my Venezuelan friend Nene, well versed in the ways of fast and *caliente* cooking, showed me the easy way to chop them:

**1.** Line up the herbs with the leaves at one end and the stubs at the other (generally, this is how they're sold).
**2.** Slice off the thicker parts of the stalk with a single cut, just below where the leaves start. Discard leafless stalk.
**3.** Fold remaining leaves in half at the middle.
**4.** Holding folded herbs tightly, cut into ¼-inch sections.

The stalk sections nearest the leaves carry flavor and texture, so it is OK to leave them in the chopped mix. But when in doubt . . . just use dried herbs.

## Wild Rice and Broccoli

A rustic dish, easy to make and great-looking on a plate.

### You need:

🖎 Saucepan

Wild or brown rice (half or full box)

Broccoli (chopped, one bag or box frozen)

Lemon juice (two dashes)

Salt, pepper, other seasonings to taste

### Preparation:

1. Cook rice according to directions on box.
2. When rice is cooked, add chopped broccoli to the mix, but try to not cover the broccoli completely while cooking (which would release acid, causing the broccoli to turn that unappealing lime-green color). Break up clumps of frozen broccoli by beating bag or box against a hard surface before adding to rice.
3. Drain excess water after broccoli has been slightly cooked (after it's been in the mix for about five minutes).
4. Add lemon juice and seasonings.
5. Best served warm, or refrigerated and reheated.

## Maize Craze

Truly piquant, this has the sweetness of corn with the tang of sun-dried tomatoes.

### You need:

🖎 Microwavable bowl or vegetable steamer

Corn (kernels, one bag frozen)

Sun-dried tomatoes (in oil, six to eight halves)

Salt, pepper, other seasonings to taste

### Preparation:

1. Microwave or steam corn.

2. Mince sun-dried tomatoes (chop enthusiastically into tiny bits).
3. Add to corn.
4. Add seasonings.
5. Mix and serve—can be reheated in a microwave or served cold.

# Teutonic Corn

A fusion of all-American corn with pickled cabbage (sauerkraut), plus chilies for extra kick.

### You need:

🏷Vegetable steamer

Corn (kernels, one bag frozen)

**Sauerkraut** (about ¼ as much by volume as the corn)

One or two whole chilies, chopped

Salt or pepper to taste

### Preparation:

1. Steam corn.
2. Add sauerkraut to mix near end of steaming.
3. Remove from heat.
4. Add chopped chilies, to taste.
5. Serve warm or refrigerated.

# Pea Garbanzo Fiesta

Full of protein, texture, and flavor.

### You need:

🏷Vegetable steamer

Peas (frozen, whole bag or box)

Garbanzo beans (one can)

Stewed tomatoes (one can)

Salsa (half a coffee cup full)

Salt, pepper, other seasonings to taste

**Preparation:**
1. Steam peas.
2. When peas are done, add garbanzo beans.
3. Separately, microwave stewed tomatoes with salsa in large serving bowl.
4. Combine cooked peas and garbanzo beans with tomato-salsa mix.
5. Best served warm (can be reheated in microwave).

## Couscous on the Loose

Couscous offers an interesting grainy texture, while chopped grapes and cooked green peppers add two surprising tastes. Couscous is in fact a processed grain, but is not without nutritional attributes.

**You need:**

Saucepan

**Couscous** (commercially prepared, one box)

Grapes (sliced in half, about a coffee cup full)

Green peppers (chopped or thinly sliced; one bag, frozen)

Salt, pepper, other seasonings to taste (including spice mix that comes in couscous package)

**Preparation:**
1. Cook couscous according to directions on box.
2. Halfway through cooking time, add chopped green peppers to mix (alternatively, steam-cook peppers separately, then add to couscous).
3. Slice grapes into halves; add to cooked couscous.
4. Add seasonings to taste.
5. Best served warm; can be reheated in the microwave.

# Grilled Vegetables

Make use of vegetables in season and a grill (indoors or outdoors) if you have one.

### You need:

🏴 **Barbecue** (optional: George Foreman–style grill)

🏴 **Barbecue** skewers (a.k.a., shish kebab sticks)—regular barbecue grill only

**Fresh vegetables**: Corn on the cob, peppers (green, red, or yellow), plum or cherry tomatoes, red onions, mushrooms, yellow squash, and zucchini

Olive oil

Salt, pepper, fresh limes or lemons

### Preparation:

1. Cut husked corn into two-inch sections.
2. Slice peppers, onions, mushrooms, squash, and zucchini into bite-sized sections.
3. Combine with tomatoes in a mixing bowl. Drizzle with olive oil, sprinkle with salt and pepper, and mix.
4. Skewer alternating vegetables: onion, tomato, squash, pepper, etc.
5. Place on grill. Squeeze lime or lemon juice onto vegetables.
6. Turn when grill marks form on bottom side (three to five minutes, depending on intensity of heat).
7. Remove from heat before grill marks cover more than 30 percent of vegetables. Remove from skewers and place into mixing bowl. Squeeze more lime or lemon juice onto vegetables.
8. Can be served warm or refrigerated. Corn may fall off the husk, or should be eaten with a fork stabbed into the core, then held to the mouth so you can nibble at the kernels.

## Tomato Potato

A hearty dish that is healthy and surprisingly green.

### You need:

🖎 Large mixing bowl, knife, and potato masher

**Sweet potatoes** (two to four, large)

Spinach (fresh, one bag or to taste)

Tomatoes (two large, sliced—stewed tomatoes from a can are an acceptable but lesser alternative)

Onion (red or yellow, one or two to taste)

Cheese (feta or cheddar, grated, about a coffee cup full)

Lemon or lime juice (two dashes)

Salt, pepper, oregano, and other seasonings to taste

Optional: sun-dried tomatoes (about ten halves, sliced into thin slivers)

### Preparation:

1. Wash sweet potatoes to remove dirt, slice in half, then microwave until cooked through. When done, slice into small chunks with skin on; place into mixing bowl.
2. Simultaneously, wash and chop spinach into bite-sized pieces.
3. Chop onions and cheese.
4. Put spinach, onion, and cheese into mixing bowl with potatoes. Toss/mix with seasonings and lemon or lime juice.
5. Add slivers of sun-dried tomatoes (optional).
6. Place slices of tomato on top of mix. Sprinkle with oregano and serve warm (can be reheated).

## Pasta (Whole Wheat or Spinach)

MAKE PASTA ACCORDING to directions on box. Separately in a saucepan, heat tomato sauce with oregano, **basil,** or **cilantro** to boil; lower heat and simmer. Pour on pasta and serve. Option: Simmer onions or other vegetables with sauce before adding to pasta. Note: This should be served warm, so you need to cook it simultaneously with the main dish (or refrigerate and reheat it).

## Simple Sweet Potatoes

TAKE TWO OR more whole, medium-sized (about the size of your fist) **sweet potatoes**, scrubbed but not peeled, place in a microwavable bowl (lubricated with butter or cooking spray). Pierce a fork through the skin to avoid an explosion while cooking, then microwave for about four to six minutes per potato. Turn over once midway through cooking.

> Note: Microwave times vary greatly by oven wattage. Allow to stand five minutes (covered) to continue to soften; serve sliced across the top lengthwise, similar to a baked potato. Flavor with butter and brown sugar, nutmeg, and/or cinnamon sprinkled on top.

## Fancy Sweet Potatoes

Note that this takes a little extra time to make (twenty to thirty minutes). Here's a recipe that is best done in an oven—an uncommon skill for most guys—but can be made in a microwave.

### You need:

Large microwavable bowl (or casserole dish, for oven baking)

Apples (three, sliced)

Orange juice or lemon juice (¼ coffee cup full)

**Sweet potatoes** (six medium-sized, sliced then cooked)

**Butter** (one whole stick–this recipe should not be made daily)

**Brown sugar** (½ coffee cup full)

**Nutmeg** (three shakes; alternatively, use cinnamon)

### Preparation:

1. Slice potatoes into bite-sized wedges; microwave in a small puddle of water (¼-inch deep) until tender. Drain water when done cooking.
2. Mix in sliced apples, juice.
3. Separately, melt butter, mix with brown sugar and nutmeg (or cinnamon), then spread over the apples and sweet potatoes.
4. Microwave for eight to twelve minutes, stir, and then nuke for another five to ten minutes. (Oven option: Bake at 400°F for 30 to 40 minutes, or until browned.)
5. Serve warm.

## MAIN DISHES

### Salmon and Dirty Corn

The great flavors (and omega-3 fatty acids) of the salmon seep into the corn and peppers for a piquant and cohesive meal.

#### You need:

 Skillet

    Salmon (two to three fillets; about five ounces each)

    Olive oil (one dash)

    Onions (yellow, two)

    Garlic (large spoonful, minced)

    Corn (frozen, one bag)

    Green peppers (frozen, one bag)

    Chili peppers to taste

    Salt and pepper to taste

    Lemon juice (one dash)

#### Preparation:

1. Stir-fry onions and garlic in oil on medium-high heat (three to six minutes).
2. Place salmon in skillet; add lemon juice. Turn after one minute, then cook for five minutes.
3. After turning fish, add corn and green peppers to skillet; season with salt and pepper.
4. Remove fish when cooked. Continue cooking corn and peppers.
5. Add chilies to corn mix. Raise heat to high. Allow corn, peppers, and onions to continue cooking, stirring frequently, until corn starts to brown.
6. Scrape dark juices from the pan when serving; drizzle over everything.

# Cracked Peppercorn Steak

You're a fancy lad if you can pull this off well. Fortunately, it's not that difficult.

### You need:
🔨 Skillet

Lean cut of meat (twelve ounces for two people): top sirloin, top loin, tenderloin, or T-bone steak

**Cracked black pepper** (or just a lot of pre-ground black pepper)

Olive oil (one dash)

Butter (four to six pats)

Old wine (for deglazing)

### Preparation:
1. Rub steaks with oil.
2. Press into crushed pepper, coating each side.
3. Sear steaks on both sides (see instructions for basic meat searing in chapter 10, page 148).
4. Stir-fry steaks in mix of butter and oil.
5. Don't overcook—cook for only five minutes each side (for cooking times, see page 178).
6. Deglaze pan: Pour wine in pan and use spatula to mix with meat juices, oil, and butter. Burn off the alcohol (it evaporates quickly).
7. Pour over steak.


SUGGESTED SIDE DISH: simple steamed vegetable—broccoli, peas, cauliflower, green beans, asparagus.

# Light Red Beans with Chicken, Oranges, and Walnuts

The bean industry promotes this recipe as a way to drive bean consumption. As well they should: the protein-to-fat ratio of this dish is a robust 44:4 for a single serving. The mix of citrus and nuts will elevate you to a new level of taste sophistication.

### You need:

🔖 Skillet or saucepan

Chicken (two whole breasts, thawed and cut into bite-sized pieces)

Onion (one large, finely chopped)

Orange juice (one coffee cup full)

Chicken broth (one coffee cup full)

Olive oil (two large spoonfuls)

Salt and pepper to taste

**Sherry** (three large spoonfuls—or substitute old wine and a little sugar)

Cinnamon (half a small spoonful)

**Cardamom** (¼ of a small spoonful)

**Cloves** (ground, ⅛ of a small spoonful)

Raisins (half a coffee cup)

Light red kidney beans (one can, drained and rinsed)

Walnuts (in pieces, half coffee cup full)

Oranges (two, peeled, free of white membranes)

**Scallions** (two big spoonfuls, thinly sliced)

### Preparation:

1. Oil skillet; heat until oil begins to "ripple."
2. Half-cook chicken breasts with salt and pepper, enough to turn both sides white (about a minute on each side). Remove and set aside on a separate plate (covered to hold in heat).
3. Add onion to skillet and cook for about five minutes until golden.
4. Reduce heat to medium and stir in orange juice, broth, sherry, cinnamon, cardamom, cloves, and raisins. Simmer, covered, for ten minutes.
5. Add beans and simmer for two minutes. Chop chicken into bite-sized pieces.

6. Add chicken pieces back to skillet, along with walnuts and orange sections, and cook for five more minutes or until the chicken is tender (and done).
7. Taste for seasoning and add more salt or pepper if necessary.
8. The sauce can be thickened by mashing some of the beans.
9. Sprinkle with scallions; serve.

Adapted from a recipe from the Bean Education & Awareness Network, originally developed by Sally and Martin Stone (*The Instant Bean*).

# CRUSHING WALNUTS

**Y**OUR MOTHER MAY have had a nut grinder; you have brute force. Since the need for crushing this softer nut arises only occasionally, a simple way to break these critters into smaller pieces is to take two plates of equal size and put a single layer of walnuts in between them. On a firm countertop, use your body weight to press down on the plates. This will break up at least half the nuts. Stir the nuts a bit and press again. You are connecting with your primal self as you make an evolved and nutritious addition to your meal.

Another technique (used by Deanna's mother) is to place nuts in a small paper lunch bag, fold over the top, and smash a large kitchen spoon against the paper bag. This may also explain why Deanna is so well behaved today.

Note: Unless you are a WWF wrestler with super-strong dinnerware, do not use the first method on almonds or other harder nuts.

# Beefnich

Your date will love the healthy greens and cabbage; you're going to love the sirloin. It's a happy coupling.

### You need:

Deep skillet

 Chopped/ground sirloin (one pound, 90 percent lean or leaner)

 Spinach (enough to "bed" two to three plates)

 Red cabbage (⅓–½ head, chopped)

 Onion (one large, chopped)

 Diced tomatoes (one can); alternatively, ⅓ jar of tomato sauce

 Oregano, salt, black pepper, and hot pepper to taste

 Parmesan cheese

### Preparation:

1. Stir-fry onion, seasonings, and sirloin for ten to fifteen minutes on medium-high heat.
2. Chop cabbage; add after ten minutes.
3. Add tomatoes/sauce after thirteen minutes (for about two minutes of cooking time).
4. Make bed of spinach on plate (option: pre-mix greens with Italian dressing or oil/vinegar or oil/lemon mix).
5. Serve on beds of spinach; top with Parmesan cheese (optional).

# Ginger's Breasts of Chicken

Simple and a touch sweet with a bouncy bite.

### You need:

Skillet

 Olive oil (enough to lightly coat the surface of the pan)

 Onions (yellow, two small or one large)

 Chicken breasts (frozen, three to five boneless/skinless)

 Green peppers (chopped and frozen, one bag)

Ginger (minced, about two large spoonfuls)

Salt, pepper, and oregano to taste

**Preparation:**

1. Sauté onions in oil for five to ten minutes on medium-high heat.
2. Add chicken to onions; raise heat to high to braise both sides (turn after two to three minutes).
3. Reduce heat; sprinkle with oregano; cover and cook chicken until done (about four to eight minutes per side).
4. Midway through cooking, add green peppers; stir occasionally.
5. Pull out one breast to test for doneness; add ginger in last minute or two of cooking.

## Turkey Chili

At the end of the day, all that most guys want in a relationship is someone who can crack open a few beers, watch TV without a lot of unrelated commentary, and enjoy a fine bowl or two of kick-butt chili. *Is that too much to ask?* See chapter 13 for a date-friendly turkey chili recipe (page 230). Serve with a green salad.

## DESSERT

A dessert has to be easy to make after the meal is done. Each of these is very easy—and is made of ingredients you will have around the house on a day-to-day basis. So in case you spaced out on planning for this date, it is simple to pull together a dessert in just a couple of minutes.

## Peanut Butter Cottage

Soften two spoonfuls of peanut butter in the microwave in a small, individual-serving bowl. It should be enough to spread around the base of the bowl. Add dollops of cold cottage cheese onto the warm peanut butter. Sprinkle one to two packets of sweetener on the cottage cheese and spread it around with a fork (take care not to mix the sweetener with the peanut butter). Add a touch of cinnamon, raisins, or a few berries for color, taste, and texture.

## Apple Peace

All you need is love, and a couple of apples, some sweetener, cinnamon, and a microwave. Slice the apple into a bowl; sprinkle with sweetener (aspartame, sugar, or honey) and cinnamon. Microwave for one or two minutes. Serve alone, or with yogurt or ice cream.

## Yin Yang Yogurt/Applesauce

On separate serving plates—one for you, one for your date—place a dollop of yogurt alongside a dollop of applesauce. With the bottom of a large spoon, spread the lower half of the left side toward the right and the upper half of the right side toward the left, creating the yin yang symbol of Taoist philosophy (it looks like the number 69). Give the rounder globs an eye with a raisin, a pinch of cinnamon, or an herb (sage, thyme, or rosemary).

## Yogurt/Peanut Butter Pull (Formal)

You can't dip your peanut butter spoon into the yogurt tub with a date. At least not on the first date. But you can replicate that great taste with separate spoons and separate bowls of yogurt. If that still seems too primitive, make a little peanut butter mound in the middle of your dessert plates, then surround it with yogurt. A few berries, raisins, or even a little glob of fruit preserves tumbling off the peanut butter mound give it a little "visual interest."

## FINISHING UP: WHEN SHOULD YOU DO THE DISHES?

AS THE HOST, IT'S clearly your job to handle all matters of clean-up, which presents a certain dilemma: Do you leave all dirty dishes in the kitchen post-meal, attending to the needs of your date? Will that leave the impression that you're a slob?

It would be very awkward, even rude, if you left your date for more than three minutes while you made your kitchen spic-and-span. Many hosts mistakenly do this, unaware that it constitutes bad manners. Instead, minimize the mess by efficiently packing dirty dishes into the sink or dishwasher and laying a nice clean towel over the table top. Perishable foods should of course be stored in the refrigerator.

The end goal of the evening is not exactly to soak your hands in Palmolive.

## GUYS ASK WHY

**Q.** I've noticed that my dates always leave some food on their plates, even when they talk about how good it is. What's up with that?
**A.** You've most likely stumbled onto a marketing issue. Some women are instructed not to appear to overindulge in public, so a rule of thumb for them is to leave a little bit of everything on the plate. Note that this rule seems to have been disregarded by some in recent years; women are rebelling against it—if they like something, they'll eat all of it. But in some rural pockets, that may still be a practice. Don't take it personally.

**Q.** How important is the atmosphere, like candles and that stuff?
**A.** Very. The mood is half the challenge. Consider what retail stores do to sell clothes, housewares, and furniture; lighting, sound, and presentation strongly affect people's willingness to buy. The analogy holds in a date-night situation.

**Q.** How can I avoid some major date-night pitfalls?
**A.** Good question. First, be ready when your date arrives. Plan ahead and give yourself at least two to three hours to make food, clean up, etc. Second, don't make the date night your first attempt at a recipe; test each

item a day or two in advance. Third, don't over-salt or over-spice. Women tend to have more sensitive taste buds than guys, so allow the salting and spicing of a dish to be a personal option (put salt and spices on the table).

**Q.** Why not just order in?

**A.** You are missing the point. You want to demonstrate you can cook, or at least take care of yourself in the kitchen on occasion. This is often on women's short list of desirable characteristics in a mate. You might cheat a little by buying prepared dips, a side dish, or a dessert, but if you make only one thing—even a green salad—make a visible production of it so your date sees you're not incompetent. You have a marketing objective as well.

# 13

# a guy's gotta barbecue

## The care and feeding of friends can be smart, too

**There's nothing like** summer, time for a guy to kick back and fire up the barbecue—the exclusive province of men in the cooking world. Half a year later, when the Super Bowl comes around, you can put the grill away and order a pizza to watch the big game with your friends.

Well, maybe. I must inform you of some news on this front:

➲ Barbecuing may be fun, but to do it right you can't exactly "kick back." It's a logistical exercise, involving a sense of timing, the science of fire, and the art of taste. Quite often, you are expected to master these things while under the influence of alcohol.

➲ The barbecue is no longer the exclusive territory of guys. The Weber Grill people took a survey of grill owners and found that female barbecuing increased by 20 percent in the three years prior to 2002. Moreover, when women put food to fire, they "take a very different approach to grilling than men." Further, a movement known as Girls at the Grill™ (www.GirlsAtTheGrill.com) claims they do it just as well—if not better—than us. The nerve. But to the Girls' credit, they've provided us with a kick-butt Basic Beer-Can Chicken recipe (it's a little complicated, but we can do it).

➲ Summer isn't the only time people barbecue: 66 percent of grillers report using the barbecue year-round.

➲ That pizza won't cut it. Super Bowl parties have become home-entertaining extravaganzas, perhaps more about the party you throw than which league champion fails to live up to the pre-game hype.

In other words, our turf has been invaded and expectations are higher. Try not to feel threatened. Instead, arm yourself with knowledge and tools, and take back the plate, grill, and buffet table.

## CHOOSING A SMART MENU

THERE WAS A TIME in our lives, perhaps college, when a quick trip to the convenience store pretty much covered it: chips and dips, hot dogs and buns, beer and soda loaded into the trunk and you were done. But beers, dogs, and chips take their toll. The party doesn't have to end, however; a smart menu can keep the good times rolling.

This chapter works on two simultaneous tracks. The first is grilling, making the assumption that you have outdoor access (yard, patio, balcony, public park) and a grill, charcoal or gas. At the same time, there are non-grilled items that are a necessary supplement; you should be able to make these things, too. Working within the healthy framework of lean meats, fruits and vegetables, whole grains, and low-fat dairy, the following is a run-down of possible menu items for your next barbecue or party:

## GRILLING ITEMS

Turkey burgers

Lean red meat: Top sirloin steak, top loin steak, tenderloin steak, T-bone steak, ground sirloin (90 percent or higher lean), pork tenderloin, or center-cut pork chops

Chicken

Chicken sausages (as a side dish—these still have a poor protein-to-fat ratio, but are healthier than other sausages)

Roast chicken

Fish

Corn on the cob

Other vegetables

## MAIN DISHES *NOT* MADE ON THE GRILL

Chili

Other soups

Roast turkey

Salmon cakes

Order-in healthy pizza

## SIDE DISHES

Salads and casseroles

Fruit combinations

## PRE-MEAL PREPARATION

IN THE INTEREST OF giving credit where credit is due, the following advice can be attributed to Weber Grill and Girls at the Grill™, gender competition issues notwithstanding.

### CHOOSE YOUR WEAPON WISELY: GAS OR CHARCOAL

A gas grill is usually the instrument of choice of committed grillers. It's a greater up-front financial commitment; in exchange, one gets a quicker and more manageable fire. Even if you're commitment-averse, give gas solid consideration because grilling can lead to very healthy food habits and even unleash previously undiscovered cooking talents.

Charcoal grills can be purchased for as little as $25, which is great for someone just starting out. More elaborate models of both types are available on the market, but this book provides recipes that are in the "basic" category; the $25 models are sufficient for six to eight people.

## TIMING IS EVERYTHING

Since in general you will cook only one or two items on the grill, make sure that all other accompanying meal items are ready to eat at the same time. Cold and room-temperature dishes are less dependent on timing, but the hot food should be as hot as possible when served. The key, then, is to make most of the food in advance. Timing the fire is equally important; start a charcoal fire about twenty minutes before you want to start cooking to allow the charcoals to get white-hot. A gas grill will take only half that time to preheat.

## GET A THERMOMETER

In the elementary approach to grilling—where the fast, high-heat, direct method is used, versus the slower-cooking indirect method—there is a tendency for the inside of the meat to be more rare than the browned outer meat. This is why thinner cuts of red meat, chicken, or fish work better than thick ones. To be absolutely certain, an instant-read meat thermometer will enable you to gauge the internal temperature of meat, which is most crucial in more complicated large dishes (whole chickens, thicker cuts of beef on the bone, etc.). The cooked temperature at the inside of ground meats should be 160°F, 170°F for poultry.

## DON'T DRY OUT THE MEAT OR VEGETABLES

Even as you try to make sure the meat is fully cooked, you have to be careful not to overcook it to the extent that it is tough and dry. Chicken is particularly vulnerable to this. Also, searing each side of a cut of meat will seal in juices. Cutting or poking into meat with a fork, or squeezing a burger down on the grill with the spatula, will force the meat's flavorful juices to drip into the fire and will dry out the meat.

## USE FRESH AND HIGH-QUALITY INGREDIENTS

A barbecue or party is a special event, one that warrants an investment of a little more time and money than daily meal preparation. Frozen meats can be used, but can also be trickier to work with because of the defrosting process. Frozen vegetables, alas, don't work as well on the grill. Your best bet for fresh vegetables is at a farmers' market or a farm stand; your second option is the grocery store (in season, they can be just as good). If you want to throw a good party, give it the extra effort.

## FIRE IT UP

THIS IS A BOOK on basics, so we will use the fast, high-heat, direct method. It is the means by which meat and vegetables are cooked directly over heat over a short period of time, versus the indirect method, which is a slower, convection-style application of heat to thicker cuts of meat (in particular, those that have bones). The only recipe in this chapter specifically employing the indirect method is the Basic Beer-Can Chicken on page 227.

Foods best made via the direct method are *boneless* steaks, fish, and chicken, plus burgers and vegetables. Each of these should be cooked evenly on both sides, requiring a single turn midway through the cooking process. An addition of mesquite or applewood chips (or wet green herbs such as rosemary) to the flame can add flavor in the smoke, which circulates into the food when the lid is left on during the grilling process.

Step by step, here's how to do it:

1. *Prepare the Food:* You can simply place raw meat on a grill and get flavor from the caramelization that occurs as the heat reacts with naturally occurring sugars. But a marinade will soften ("denature") tissue with its acidity (marinades are a combination of oil, spices, and acidic elements such as wine, vinegar, citric juice, and even yogurt). Marinades are sold commercially prepared (vinegary salad dressings also work well), but you can make your own with as little as vinegar, an equal amount of olive oil, and a few spices. Fish and other tender meats should be marinated for less than an hour; chicken and beef can be marinated for one to four hours.

    Vegetables should be washed and cut as desired. Cut slices wide enough that they will not fall through the grill, or will hold together on a skewer. Some of the best grilling vegetables are fresh peppers (green, orange, yellow, red), onions, pear and cherry tomatoes, potatoes, and mushrooms. Green and yellow beans, beefsteak tomatoes, squash, eggplant, and zucchini also work well if you can keep them from falling through the grill (use greased aluminum foil or a metal pan). Regardless of whether you cook on skewers or simply on the grill, a light coating of olive oil and seasonings will keep the vegetables moist and tasty.

2. *Prepare the Grill:* Gas grill prep is so easy I won't insult your intelligence to describe it here. But charcoal is another matter. You want the heat of white-hot ash on the charcoal briquettes (white-hot is hotter than glowing red). Timing is critical because it takes about twenty minutes from lighting to achieve that level of heat, but after the briquettes reach that level they will burn down and you'll begin to get a lower-intensity heat (you can boost it if you add some briquettes to the already-lit fire). The bottom line is that this is an inexact process; you'll need to closely monitor progress on the grill.

3. *Grill It:* Once the optimum level of heat has been achieved, begin placing food on the grill. Cooking times vary by the cut of meat and your own preferences for doneness, but all grilled items should require fifteen minutes or less over direct heat.

4. *Serve It:* As the meat or grilled vegetables are cooking, begin to get pre-made items (salads, casseroles) out and ready for service, along with dinnerware (plates, utensils, paper towels or napkins).

# A BASIC REVIEW, ALPHABETIZED

**E**LIZABETH KARMEL HAS graciously allowed us to borrow the following (slightly adapted) from her Web site, www.GirlsAtTheGrill.com.

**A**ccurate instant-read meat thermometer will take the guesswork out of *testing for doneness.*

**B**urned barbecue is bad barbecue.

**C**lose lid while cooking.

**D**irect cooking method: When the only thing that comes between your steak and the fire is the grill grate.

**E**xtinguish flare-ups by closing the lid—never use a water bottle.

**F**uel. Make sure you have enough charcoal or that your gas tank is full.

**G**ray-ash-covered charcoal means you're ready to cook.

**H**ave fun. It's about the fun (but that doesn't negate the idea of serving smart food).

**I**ndirect cooking method: More like a convection oven, when the heat is directed around and over the food with a metal pan in between food and fire.

**J**ust grill it. Brush with olive oil (sparingly), sprinkle with salt, and the food is ready to grill.

**K**eep the grill clean by using a brass bristle brush to clean the cooking grates.

**L**ocking long-handled tongs are much easier to use than traditional barbecue tongs.

**M**ake sure your "mess is in place." Be organized.

**N**uke the chicken in juice or water; there's less chance for *salmonella* to survive and you're more likely to serve moist meat.

**O**live oil. Put a thin coating on vegetables before grilling.

**P**reheat your grill—especially with charcoal, be sure to start the fire at least twenty minutes in advance of when you want to start grilling.

**Q**uestions? Don't be afraid to ask your guests for help.

**R**est. Let the meat rest for five to ten minutes before slicing and serving.

**S**alt. Use only kosher or sea salt, because it is inexpensive and lacks additives, and its flakes dissolve quickly.

**T**urn only once halfway through cooking time.

**U**se barbecue sauce only during the last twenty minutes of cooking time.

**V**ents. Keep them open to keep the fire burning.

**W**ash your hands and wash platters between raw and cooked stages to prevent cross-contamination (very important—it's not nice to make your guests sick).

**X**-tra fast: how you sear juices into meat, placing the cut near the hottest part of the fire (or just turning up the flame) for one to two minutes on each side, then lowering heat to cook all the way through.

**Y**ummy juices. Keep them in the food—use tongs instead of a fork (piercing the food allows the juices to run out).

**Z**ucchini. Grill beyond corn and potatoes—*many of us believe that vegetables taste better when grilled.*

# BARBECUE AND OTHER FOODS FOR ENTERTAINING

## APPETIZERS

Because barbecues and parties are more of a journey than a destination, you will probably spend a portion (one-half to two-thirds) of the affair working on the food that others will eat. In fact, the eating part may take mere minutes after hours of preparation and cooking. And guests will expect food the minute they arrive, which is why someone invented appetizers—little foods to tide us over until the main stuff is done.

Appetizers are historically fatty, but health consciousness in recent years has brought about several better-for-you innovations. Here are a few ideas that are simple to execute and appropriately tasty.

### Half Hard-Boiled Eggs

This is the easier version of deviled eggs. Hard-boil three eggs for every two people in attendance. When done and cooled, remove the shell and slice in half lengthwise, being sure to split the yolk between both halves. Arrange on a plate or platter, then drip one or two drops of lemon (or lime) juice and hot sauce on each egg half. Or try mustard, horseradish, or paprika.

### Baby Carrots, Grapes, Crackers, and Cheddar Cheese

None of these items cook well on a grill, so make them your pre-meal snack. Arrange each on a large serving platter or plate, providing a small knife for slicing the cheese (try a low-fat cheddar or goat cheese). Provide small salad plates for guests.

### Vegetable Tray

If you're not grilling vegetables for the main meal, you can serve finger-sized pieces of fresh peppers, perhaps with pepperoncini and hummus dip.

### Shrimp Not on the Barbie

Most shrimp sold in stores are cooked and ready to eat (the pink kind). Just put them on a plate or bed of ice (don't let them hang out in warm air too long) alongside lemon slices and a bowl of cocktail sauce.

### Taco Corn Chips and Salsa

OK, so it's not very creative. It's still a pretty popular favorite, and the salsa is a healthy addition to any meal (it sure beats the mayo-based dips with ruffled potato chips we used to eat as kids). See if you can find baked corn chips to substitute for the standard fried versions. This appetizer goes well with beer.

### Coleslaw

Slaw is a great picnic food because it holds its crunch in the heat, provides a great balance to meat, and is recognized by people in the know as very healthy when made without or with minimum mayonnaise (in the vinegar-based German style). How to do it: Chop red or green cabbage; separately, heat a little oil, a lot of vinegar, vegetables, and spices (including mustard, peppers, chopped onions, and whatever else you like) in a skillet. Drop the chopped cabbage into the hot dressing, remove from heat after a few seconds, and cool in a refrigerator.

### Salmon Cakes

With canned salmon, mince and mash the fish, then mix with equal amounts (by volume) of minced vegetables and spices (green peppers, tomatoes, onions, and paprika, cilantro, or basil, for example). Mix in a few large spoonfuls of egg whites and a handful of bread crumbs, then form into small cakes and fry in a skillet at medium-high heat for three to four minutes on each side. Serve hot or reheated in the microwave, with cocktail sauce.

## GRILLING ITEMS

While a barbecue almost seems to require the use of red meat, a mixed crowd might include an individual or two who is either vegetarian or limits meat consumption to fish and chicken. In general, non-red meats also will be lower in fat. That's why alternatives such as ground turkey, chicken, and fish are included here; you can substitute ground beef (95 percent lean) in most recipes.

## Turkey Burgers

Turkey burgers have achieved wide acceptance as an alternative to beef burgers; in fact, many guests can't tell the difference. They can be purchased prepared and frozen, but if you want to make your own it's pretty simple and uses ingredients already on your shopping list. Assume guests will eat two burgers each; this recipe yields only four burgers, so multiply recipe ingredients by the number of people you are serving. A word of caution here: Ground turkey sometimes includes the skin ground in with the meat, making it a poor nutritional choice (it's actually higher in fat and calories than burgers made from most ground beef). So, be careful when buying ground turkey—look for the word *lean*, ideally 85 percent lean or higher.

### You need:

Fresh ground turkey (1 pound, at least 85 percent lean)

Onion (½ coffee cup full, chopped)

One egg or equivalent egg white

Garlic (small spoonful, minced)

Ketchup (¼ coffee cup full)

Pepper (three to four dashes)

Oregano (large spoonful)

Optional: chopped fresh herbs (**cilantro**, **basil**, or **rosemary**)—if you are gril-ing the burgers immediately, not if you are preparing them several hours in advance (herbs either lose their flavor or can turn bitter over time)

### Preparation:

1. Combine turkey, onion, eggs, garlic, ketchup, pepper, oregano, and optional fresh herbs in a bowl, mixing with a fork. Form into four burgers, approximately 3½" in diameter.
2. Grill turkey burgers five to six minutes per side until meat is no longer pink in center (165°F is reached on meat thermometer).
3. Serve on whole-grain buns alongside standard condiments (onions, relish, mustard, lettuce, etc.).

## Steak (Top Sirloin, Top Loin, Tenderloin, T-Bone)

As elsewhere in this book, the leanest cuts of red meat are recommended. Cooking times are short because there is less fat to keep the steak moist and tender.

### You need:

Selected cut of beef (approximately one inch thick)

Olive oil (enough for a light coating on both sides of each steak)

Salt and pepper to taste

### Preparation:

1. Let steaks stand at room temperature for about twenty minutes.
2. Apply olive oil to steaks, then salt/pepper to taste (don't overdo it if you are restricting your salt intake.
3. Sear each side on grill (one minute each); push coals into a higher pile on half the grill to achieve a temporarily higher heat.
4. Grill steaks for about five to six minutes on each side (with the coals evenly spread out).

# NUKING THE CHICKEN

**S**AY "MICROWAVED CHICKEN" to an experienced chef and you're likely to get a disapproving look. Fortunately, you do not care. And some of the experts back us up. One reason most cookbooks don't suggest nuked food is due to the variability between the cooking power of different microwave ovens, (700 watts? 1,500 watts?), which prevents specific cooking instructions.* Another objection on the part of the culinary cognoscenti is how conventional cooking will brown the edges of the meat, something that doesn't happen in a microwave. But guys are free of such constrained thinking. For the most part, the microwave satisfies our need for immediate gratification. And it cuts down on dirty dishes, enabling us to prepare and sometimes eat meals from a single bowl. Commercial browning sauces are available, if that matters to you.

"Microwaving is a safe and acceptable way to prepare chicken dishes," says Bill Roenigk, vice president of the National Chicken Council. "Some people prefer to cook it into a sauce. And some people microwave chicken before putting it on an outdoor grill to speed up the process." And Bill should know his chickens.

With whatever method you use, always test for doneness (no pink meat in the middle), and allow the chicken to stand for a few minutes after nuking to make sure the bacteria is dead.

*All recipes in this book were developed for a 1,500-watt microwave.

## Chicken (Boneless/Skinless)

Boneless and skinless chicken breasts are the simplest to make, including both those purchased fresh and your standard frozen varieties. The trick is to cook the chicken adequately without overcooking.

### You need:
Chicken breasts (estimate two per person)
Olive oil (enough for a light coating over each breast)
Salt and pepper to taste

### Preparation:
1. If starting with frozen chicken breasts, microwave on "defrost" according to directions on microwave oven. Alternatively, thaw in cold tap water in refrigerator for one to three hours before beginning the cooking process. Rinse thawed breasts in cold water and pat dry with paper towels.
2. Apply olive oil to both sides of each breast; season with salt and pepper.
3. Microwave approximately two to four minutes per chicken breast, until outside is no longer pink.
4. Grill breasts approximately three to five minutes per side over fire until done (no pink inside). Test one breast by cutting in half to check for doneness.

## Basic Beer-Can Chicken (Whole Roasting Chicken)*

Grilling method: Indirect/medium heat

### You need:

One four-to-five-pound roasting chicken (recommended: Amish or kosher)

One twelve-ounce can of beer

Dry spice rub (three large spoonfuls—dry rub is a mix of spices, your own concoction or as sold packaged)

Olive oil

Kosher salt and freshly ground pepper

### Preparation:

1. Because this requires the indirect heating method, you will need a grill that is large enough to move white-hot ashes to the side or a metal heat-deflector placed under the chicken; gas grills that have different settings for various sections of the grill also enable this. An indirect heat source is slower but applies more uniform heat to the chicken.

2. Remove neck and giblets (innards) and pat dry with paper towels. Brush chicken all over with oil and season with two large spoonfuls dry rub and salt and pepper. Set aside.

3. Open beer can, drink about ¼ cup of the beer, and make an extra hole in the top of the can with a church key can opener. Sprinkle the remaining tablespoon of the dry rub inside the beer can. Place the beer can in the center of the cooking grate and move the legs of the chicken apart so the body cavity slides over the top of the beer can. The chicken will appear to be "sitting" on the grate. Cover for cooking purposes and so that guests are not made to feel uncomfortable with this image.

4. Cook chicken for sixty to ninety minutes or until the internal temperature registers 165°F in the breast area and 180°F in the thigh. Remove from grill and let rest for ten minutes before carving.

**Danger! Danger, Will Robinson!** When removing the chicken from the grate, be careful not to spill the contents of the beer can, as it will be very hot. Grab the bottom of the beer can with a pair of locking tongs and place it on a platter or cutting board to cool.

*Recipe used with permission from Girls at the Grill™: ©2002, Girls at the Grill™ (Elizabeth Karmel)

## Fish

Salmon remains at the top of our favorites among fish; however, you should feel free to experiment with other types. The challenge with many types of fish is keeping them from falling apart and into the fire; a foil layer on the grill or a foil pan helps. Steaks or fillets work best.

### You need:

Salmon (chinook or coho, eight to sixteen ounces of steak per person; best to get fresh)
Olive oil (enough for a light coating on the fish)
Salt

### Preparation:

1. Salt both sides of salmon steaks.
2. Fire up the grill and achieve a medium-hot temperature (approximately three inches above the fire).
3. Cook fish for approximately five minutes, then turn. Continue cooking five more minutes or so until fish gets flaky (breaks up easily).
4. Serve with lemon or lime wedges.

For another salmon recipe, Salmon and Dirty Corn, see chapter 12.

## Corn on the Cob

I prefer corn boiled on the stove, but the unhusked cobs on a grill seem to hold more romance for many people. Following is what I've learned from my friends.

**You need:**

> **Corn on the cob** (husk still on, about two to three per person)
> A tub or kettle to soak the cobs in
> Butter and salt

**Preparation:**

1. Pull back husks without detaching them; remove the corn silk. Return husks to original position, perhaps binding them at the cob tip by tying with a single husk leaf.
2. Soak the corn in water (submerged) for a half-hour.
3. Place on grill (medium heat, about three to five inches from coals), turning three or four times until kernels are tender. Test one cob for doneness.
4. Serve with butter and salt, allowing guests to flavor according to their preferences.

## Grilled Vegetables

Grilled vegetables capture the essence of fire applied to food with the caramelization of naturally occurring (plant) sugars. And as you know by now, they're really good for you. The use of skewers is recommended, and is particularly useful for smaller items such as cherry tomatoes and mushrooms that would otherwise fall through the grill into the fire; larger pieces (e.g., halves of green peppers) could be grilled directly without skewers to hold them together.

**You need:**

> **Skewers** (wood or metal, sold in various sizes to accommodate different grill dimensions)
> Mixing bowl

Grillable vegetables: Fresh peppers (green, yellow, red, orange), onions, mushrooms, tomatoes (smaller pear and cherry tomatoes work best on skewers), **zucchini, eggplant**

Olive oil

Salt and pepper to taste

### Preparation:

1. Soak wood skewers in water to fireproof them.
2. Wash and slice vegetables into bite-sized pieces (tomatoes should remain whole).
3. In a large bowl, drizzle olive oil over the vegetables and toss; add salt and pepper.
4. Skewer vegetables in alternating fashion (e.g., pepper, onion, tomato, mushroom, zucchini, pepper . . .).
5. Place on grill, turning two to three times after approximately three to four minutes on each turn.
6. Remove from grill, laying skewers onto a service platter.

## NON-GRILLED MAIN DISHES

## Turkey Chili

Like turkey burgers, turkey chili has found mainstream acceptance and is almost indistinguishable from beef chili because of the strong flavors of the other ingredients.

### You need:

🔖 Large skillet

🔖 Second skillet or saucepan

Turkey (lean ground; one pound for every three people)

Olive oil (one large spoonful)

Onion (one to two large, chopped)

Fresh pepper (one to two, chopped into bite-sized pieces)

Salt and pepper to taste

Chili (any form: powder, dried, or sauce, to taste)

Garlic (large spoonful, minced)

Water (two coffee cups full)

Tomatoes (stewed, one to two cans)

Oregano (one to two large spoonfuls)

Kidney beans (one to two cans, drained and rinsed)

Sugar (one packet or half a small spoonful)

Fresh cilantro (one bunch, chopped)

### Preparation:

1. Brown ground turkey (on medium heat) with garlic and onions in skillet for about ten minutes, stirring frequently and breaking up chunks of meat. Remove from heat.
2. In the second skillet or saucepan, stir-fry fresh peppers with salt and pepper for about five minutes.
3. Add chili and water, stirring constantly until mix thickens (less than five minutes).
4. Combine two skillets into one, adding tomatoes, oregano, beans, and sugar. Simmer at least forty-five minutes. Add cilantro at the end.

# Roast Chicken

Sure, you can pretty much just pop these babies into the oven and heat at 350°F for one hour. But a little added citrus and ginger flavoring is easy and makes it much more savory.

### You need:

🏴 Oven

🏴 **Chicken roasting pan**

🏴 **Vegetable/cheese grater**

Chicken (one whole **roaster**, about five pounds)

Zest* of one lemon, then cut the lemon into quarters

Zest of one orange, then cut orange into quarters

Ginger root (peeled and grated, three large spoonfuls)

Salt and pepper to taste

Olive oil (five large spoonfuls)

Lemon juice (four large spoonfuls)

Orange juice (one coffee cup full)

**Honey** (three large spoonfuls)

### Preparation:

1. Heat oven to 350°F.
2. Rub the outside of the chicken with one of the lemon quarters.
3. In a small bowl, stir together the lemon and orange zests and one large spoonful of the grated ginger. Rub this mixture evenly into the cavity (inside) of the chicken. Put the other lemon quarters and the orange quarters inside the bird.
4. Place the chicken on a rack in a roasting pan. Sprinkle it with salt and pepper.
5. In the same (now-empty) small bowl, combine the olive oil, lemon and orange juices, honey, and the remaining two large spoonfuls of ginger. Mix well.
6. Place chicken in the oven and roast.
7. Baste (brush or pour over top) with citrus juice mixture at least four times during cooking, until juices run clear when thigh is pierced with a knife (about one hour).
8. Transfer to platter and let rest ten to fifteen minutes. Carve chicken.

*Zest is the highly acidic result of using a cheese grater on the outer skin of citrus; be careful not to get the "pith," the bitter white inside of the citrus skin.

# Roast Turkey

There may come a Thanksgiving or other holiday when you are hosting a dinner on your own. No need to panic; cooking a turkey is pretty easy—just be sure to remove the paper bag of giblets (organ meats and neck) from the inside. And, contrary to its name, stuffing should not be made stuffed inside the turkey (it prevents thorough cooking, making the survival of bacteria in the roasting process possible). The stove-top variety of stuffing works fine. As for the other dishes, you can make them yourself, but most guests are happy to help out.

### You need:

🔖 Roasting pan (the disposable kind helps with the clean-up process)
🔖 Aluminum foil

✍Meat thermometer

**Turkey** (whole, fresh, around fifteen pounds)

Olive or vegetable oil (one coffee cup full)

Salt and pepper, to taste

Commercially prepared seasoning mix, such as herb/onion

## Preparation:

1. Preheat oven to 325°F.
2. Remove giblet bag. Rinse turkey with cold water inside and out. Dry turkey with a paper towel.
3. Rub olive or vegetable oil onto the skin and inside the turkey. Add salt, pepper, and seasonings to both sides of the turkey.
4. Place turkey breast-side down (so the legs are pointing down and the backbone is facing up) on a V-rack inside a shallow roasting pan. Mold aluminum foil tightly to the turkey.
5. Place turkey in oven and cook for about 3½ hours (fifteen minutes per pound).
6. When there is about a half-hour left to cook, remove the foil and flip the turkey breast-side-up to brown.
7. The turkey is done when the meat thermometer inserted into the thickest part of the thigh (not touching the bone) reads about 180°F.
8. Allow to stand for about twenty minutes before carving.
9. Drippings from the turkey should be saved; pour off the clear (fat) layer for tasty gravy (the darker portion is more protein than fat).

## Order-In Healthier Pizza

If friends just stop by—or you fail miserably at the intended meal (through no fault of your own, of course)—you can still order a pizza and make it a semi-healthy meal. Order it with half of the cheese, no meat toppings, and plenty of vegetables (tomato slices, onions, green peppers). Then make a bean dish alongside a green salad. Serve a dessert of fruit and yogurt.

## Wild West Pizza

Make your own pizza? Sure, just substitute pita or another flat bread for traditional dough and you've got yourself a rootin', tootin' bean and ham dish appropriate for an appetizer or main meal. The per-serving protein to fat ratio could make you strong enough to rustle cattle, 26 grams of protein to 8 grams of fat—well within the target of 3:1.

### You need:
🥄 Skillet

Cooking spray

Low-fat ham (sliced, two ounces cut into ¼-inch strips)

Red kidney or pinto beans (one can)

Corn (one coffee cup full)

Green onions (sliced, including tops, ½ coffee cup full;
   substitute other onions if desired)

Fresh pepper (green or red, chopped, ½ coffee cup full)

Mozzarella cheese (four to six ounces part-skim, shredded)

Oregano (one small spoonful)

Pita or other flat breads (four)

Tomatoes (two medium, chopped)

### Preparation:
1. Spray small skillet with cooking spray; heat on medium until hot.
2. Add ham; cook over medium heat until browned and crisp (two to three minutes).
3. Coarsely mash beans; stir in corn, onions, bell pepper, half the cheese, and oregano.
4. Season with salt and pepper to taste.
5. Spread mixture on bread.
6. Top with tomatoes.
7. Bake on cookie sheets (or aluminum foil on oven racks) at 400°F until hot through, about ten minutes.
8. Sprinkle with remaining cheese; bake until cheese is melted, two to three minutes.

Adapted from a recipe by the Bean Education & Awareness Network. Reprinted with permission.

### *Non-Grilled Side Dishes (Salads and Casseroles)*

An easy barbecue or party is one where the side dishes are one-bowl wonders: mostly casseroles, made up of Main Stuff, Flavor, and Crunch. Most can be made ahead and served chilled or at room temperature.

## Basic Green Salad

See chapter 12 for a simple green salad and simple homemade oil-and-vinegar salad dressings.

## Cold Chicken Salad

In case you need to make a dish ahead of time, this could be it. A chicken salad can also serve as an alternative for guests who avoid red meat. The chicken could be cooked on the grill or made inside by traditional methods.

### You need:

Chicken (four breasts, boneless skinless, cooked and cubed)

Arugula or other greens, like spinach (about enough to fill a soccer ball)

Green grapes (one large bunch, washed and individually chopped into halves)

Sun-dried tomatoes (minced, about ⅔ coffee cup full)

Fat-free Caesar dressing (½–1 coffee cup full, to taste)

Couscous (entire contents from a commercially prepared box)

Parmesan cheese

### Preparation:

1. Cook chicken according to your preferred method (microwaved, stir-fried, or on the barbecue).
2. Cut chicken into bite-sized pieces.
3. Cook couscous according to instructions on box.
4. Wash and chop arugula (or other greens).
5. Mince sun-dried tomatoes (into one- to two-inch slivers).
6. Halve grapes.
7. Mix everything together in a single bowl; add salad dressing.
8. Refrigerate and serve cold, with Parmesan cheese.

## Honey-Orange Bean and Vegetable Slaw

A lot of great stuff combined into a rich salad. With full-fat dressing, the protein-to-fat ratio is 3:2; use a fat-free dressing and that ratio will improve.

### You need:

Red kidney or large lima beans (one can)

Navy or garbanzo beans (one can)

Pinto or red kidney beans (one can)

Red cabbage (pickled, sixteen-ounce jar)

Broccoli florets (fresh, or half a bag of frozen chopped broccoli)

Raisins (half a coffee cup full)

Dried apricots (sliced, half a coffee cup full)

Walnuts (chopped, half a coffee cup full)

French dressing (one coffee cup full)

Optional: Substitute lemon or lime juice for French dressing, dried cranberries for dried apricots, or pecans or pine nuts for walnuts

### Preparation:

1. Combine all ingredients in a large bowl.
2. Chill or serve at room temperature.

Adapted from a recipe by the Bean Education & Awareness Network. Reprinted with permission.

## Four Bean Salad

Some people think they're too sophisticated for this dish. I don't give a rat's caboose about what they think, since it's perhaps the healthiest food you'll find on a picnic table (you gotta also love the Flavor and Crunch).

### You need:

🔖 Vegetable steamer

🔖 Large mixing bowl

Canned beans (one can each of garbanzo, kidney, and black beans—three cans total)

Fresh beans (a heaping handful of both yellow and green)

Italian dressing (fat-free, ⅔ coffee cup full); optional substitutions are other types of dressings

Fresh herbs (cilantro, basil, dill, rosemary, or thyme, to taste, chopped)

### Preparation:

1. Wash and cut fresh beans (into one- to two-inch sections).
2. Steam fresh beans (or just drop them into a kettle of boiling water for a minute, a process called "blanching"); do not cook past the point where the bean breaks crisply.
3. Mix with all other ingredients in mixing bowl.
4. Chill before serving for at least thirty minutes.

## Brazilian Black Bean Bake

Carmen Miranda wore fruit on her head. You can put bananas and mangoes on top of this bean dish if you have *deux testiculo*.

### You need:

Oven-tempered casserole dish

Onions (two coffee cups full, chopped)

Chilis (two large spoonfuls, minced)

Ginger (two to four small spoonfuls, minced)

Black beans (four cans, rinsed and drained)

Diced tomatoes (two cans)

Honey (½ coffee cup full)

Brown sugar (½ coffee cup full)

Thyme (small spoonful, dried)

Salt (one small spoonful)

Mango (½ coffee cup full, cubed from jar)

Banana (½ coffee cup full, sliced)

### Preparation:

1. Mix all ingredients except mango and banana in a casserole dish.
2. Bake at 350°F, covered, for thirty minutes.
3. Uncover and bake to desired thickness, about one hour.

4. Mix mango and banana.

5. Spoon mango and banana mixture onto beans before serving.

Adapted from a recipe by the Bean Education & Awareness Network. Reprinted with permission.

## Cheaters Potato Salad

Buy prepared potato salad (in the deli or in cans)—but get the German style, which is significantly lower in fat because it's made with vinegar, not mayonnaise. Add a form of protein—chunks of ham, a couple cans of kidney or black beans, or perhaps even chopped chicken (cooked). Then add chopped herbs (cilantro, dill, basil) and/or chopped greens. Tell people it was your grandma's recipe from the old country.

## Cool Red Salad

Fruits, vegetables, and cheese in the same dish? Just try it.

### You need:
Red cabbage (⅓ head, chopped)
One handful of raisins
One large chopped apple
Two handfuls of cheddar or goat cheese, chopped into little pieces
Dash of lemon juice
Six spoonfuls of sugar/sweetener
Cinnamon

### Preparation:
1. Steam the cabbage in a deep skillet in the lemon juice (add a little water) for ten to fifteen minutes.
2. Add apple bits, raisins, cheese, cinnamon, and sugar; toss.
3. Chill before serving for at least thirty minutes

## Peanut Butter Cabbage

It doesn't get any weirder than this (with thanks to Thailand for showing us what a great combination spices and peanuts can be).

### You need:
Cabbage (½ head, chopped)
Lemon juice (two dashes)
Tabasco sauce (a dash or two)
Peanut butter (two to three tablespoons)

### Preparation:
1. Cook cabbage in lemon juice and Tabasco sauce in a deep skillet for about ten to fifteen minutes.
2. Add peanut butter; toss.
3. Serve hot.

## Fruit Combinations

LET OTHERS BRING the ice cream. Watermelon is always a good picnic food, but make it a little more interesting with one of the following:

## Nutty Banana

The bananas might go mushy, but the nuts keep things crunchy. The third ingredient is purely optional, so I suggest whatever is in season.

### You need:
Bananas (four to six, peeled and sliced)
Nuts (peanuts, crushed walnuts, or crushed almonds)
One more fruit (strawberries, blueberries, peaches, pears, or anything else of
    your choosing)
Sweetener to taste
Cinnamon to taste
Lemon juice or orange juice (two to three large spoonfuls) to help reduce the
    oxidation (browning) of the bananas

**Preparation:**

1. Mix all ingredients in a bowl.
2. Serve chilled or warmed in a saucepan on the stove, and pour over ice cream.

# Marshmallow Citrus

Similar to the ambrosia your mother made, this refreshing dessert is ideal on a hot day.

**You need:**

Mixing bowl

Serving bowl

**Mandarin** or **clementine oranges**, sectioned (about three small oranges)

Pineapple chunks, drained (two coffee cups full)

**Flaked coconut** (sprinkle on top only, about four large spoonfuls)

**Miniature marshmallows** (two coffee cups full)

Yogurt (low-fat plain or vanilla, one coffee cup full)

Sweetener (one small spoonful)

**Maraschino cherries** (enough to sprinkle around top of bowl)

**Preparation:**

1. Mix the fruit, sweetener, and coconut thoroughly in mixing bowl.
2. Fold in the yogurt and marshmallows.
3. Transfer to decorative serving bowl, cover with plastic wrap, and refrigerate up to twenty-four hours.
4. Sprinkle coconut flakes on top.
5. Right before serving, garnish with a few maraschino cherries.

One last point: Barbecues and other parties are a great opportunity to enlist your guests in your cooking ventures. They might have some great ideas. Because when you think about it, part of eating smart is to get others to do some of the work for you. I do it all the time.

Good luck—and make it clear to your female guests that they're not taking over our territory just yet.

# PART IV

# GET OUTTA THE HOUSE

## MAKING YOUR own

meals at home will almost always be more nutritious, time-efficient, and economical than eating out. But to suggest you will or should *always* eat at home is pure fantasy. Eating out is the Big Reality of modern life. Big, as in how meals prepared outside the home constitute between 34 and 45 percent of what we eat in total; and Reality, as in how eating out is a matter of making do with circumstances beyond your control. Remember that research tells us meals outside the home contain 55 percent more calories on average. Eat out all the time and chances are you'll become really big.

The good news is that the food industry provides more options than ever. You *should* be able to find food that is both smart and satisfying. The bad news is that there is lots of room to trip up, times when you might think you're eating smart when in fact you are not, or healthful choices that simply aren't there when you are hungry.

You live a busy life, and consequently you often eat outside the home. Your eyes scan the roadways and storefronts, or you think about going to a vending machine near your workplace, or a snack shop or fast-food joint nearby. Time and proximity have a way of creating limits.

You may be eating with other people who have a different set of objectives than yours, such as the "working lunch." Or in a group where a vocal member can't have anything but pizza, or someone else insists on trying the hot new place. Group-think rarely takes nutrition into consideration. There are also the holiday dinners with family, which offer a preponderance of processed carbohydrates, dripping with butter. That's Reality. You simply can't call all the shots in such situations.

The principle is not very different from the famous serenity prayer: Control what you can, accept what you can't, and practice the wisdom of eating just a little smarter at home the day after you eat a slice of Aunt Edna's prize-winning rhubarb-strawberry pie.

# 14

# a guy's gotta eat out

## Guys eat out more than anyone else—all the more reason to do it right

**About half of** your food dollars are spent outside the home. It's a plain fact of modern life—Americans dole out $222 billion in restaurants each year, $118 million of that in "QSRs" (quick-service restaurants—a.k.a. fast food). The convenience culture is integral to our way of life.

And guys like us love it. According to the Center for Science in the Public Interest (*Restaurant Confidential*, Workman Publishing, 2002), younger men are more likely to eat outside the home than other demographic categories. "Thirty-four percent of our calories are consumed outside the home; this figure rises to 45 percent for men in the 18–39-year-old age bracket," say authors Michael F. Jacobson, Ph.D. and Jayne G. Hurley, R.D.

You must resolve to beat the averages. Don't be a victim of statistics; since the life span of the average man is shorter than that of the average woman, you have plenty of reason and incentive to eat at home. But even with the best of efforts, you will still eat about a quarter of your meals out. Your plan, then, is simple: Eat smart in restaurants, while traveling, when you are a guest in someone else's home, or when you need a quick bite.

In other words, if you can't beat 'em, join 'em—in the smartest way possible. Want some quick tips? Here are some simple rules of thumb to guide you through most situations:

- **Fast food:** Chicken, turkey, and (believe it or not) roast beef almost always trump everything else—including tuna salad (which usually is loaded with mayonnaise). The restaurant industry has found ways to screw up otherwise healthy fish and fowl by breading, battering, and frying it, and applying tons of mayonnaise. Study, pay attention, and ask questions—and substitute mustard, lemon juice, and/or hot sauce for mayonnaise.
- **Finer dining:** Order the (good) things you don't make yourself. If you don't often cook red meat, get one of the leaner cuts of beef: top sirloin steak, top loin steak, tenderloin steak, or T-bone steak.
- **Menu words to *like*:** Grilled, steamed, stir-fried (sometimes), tomato sauce, and tomato broth.
- **Menu words to *dislike*:** Fried, refried, deep-fried, crispy, cream sauce, butter, breaded, batter-dipped, and lightly coated. Fried potatoes (French fries, chips, etc.) in particular are a deal killer at any meal.
- **Breakfasts out:** Eggs (whites only), not waffles or pancakes; whole-wheat toast, not white, rye, or even pumpernickel (dark coloration of a bread does not mean it's made from the complete grain). Croissants are made from refined flour and have more fat than breads, bagels, and burrito wraps—sorry, France, but we don't need any.

⊃ **Travel:** Most domestic flights no longer offer real meals, so pack your own meals and/or snacks or be sure to eat before you leave. On the highway, pack food but also learn how to make the best choices at the fast-food chains, diners, and truck stops that dominate highway exits.

⊃ **Hotel (extended stay):** Stock the mini-refrigerator with orange juice, low-fat yogurt, fresh fruit (apples, bananas, peaches, pears, strawberries, oranges, etc.), and other smart snack foods. (You can even make instant oatmeal in the coffee maker.) In most urban areas and many suburbs there are either greengrocers (in New York, in particular) or healthier-food chain grocers; ask the hotel concierge or your business colleagues for suggestions.

Keep those tips in mind and you should be able to navigate the big bad food world outside your house. The rest of this chapter provides specific ideas on how to eat smart at different times of the day, in various types of restaurants, and in common situations (post-workout, working lunches, social events) that may well constitute a large portion of your eating life.

# BLAME THE FRENCH (AS USUAL)

**J**UST IN CASE you missed the point, French fries are the bane of a guy's existence. Why?

- On average, Americans eat fifty pounds of fries a year—and guys skew higher than average. Fifty pounds.
- Think about it: Why do restaurants serve French fries with everything? Because they are cheap fillers (the same with the bread). Your health is not their concern.
- Why do French fries taste good? Anything containing that much fat, starch, and salt usually does. It's a quick fix that also digests quickly and causes your blood sugar to shoot upwards.
- Most beneficial nutrients in potatoes lie just below the skin. Most fries have that part peeled off.
- The potassium in a regular order of French fries—most often cited as the redeeming nutrient—at major fast-food chains is equivalent to the amount in roughly one large bite of a banana.

- If you cut three supersize orders of McDonald's French fries a week from your diet, you'll reduce your calorie intake by 95,160 calories per year, which could translate into **27** pounds of lost body weight.
- The French are thin, but that's because they eat everything in smaller quantities than we do. And their crinkly deep-fried pota- toes (*pommes frites*) are a treat for a special occasion for them, eaten in balance with other heart-healthy foods (such as goat cheese, tomatoes stir-fried in olive oil, and red wine). Some Americans eat a bag of fries every day.

## EAT YOUR WAY THROUGH THE DAY

THE RESTAURANT INDUSTRY REFERS to our meals as "day parts"—that is, times when we eat breakfast, lunch, and dinner. We tend to eat different types of food in different types of places for each.

### BREAKFAST

Consumer research has found that people's intentions to eat healthy are best in the morning—we like to start the day on the right foot. Those good intentions get scant support from the hospitality industry.

➲ *Biggest pitfalls:* Fast-food egg-sandwich meals; donuts; carb-heavy but protein-deficient waffles, pancakes, and French toast; bacon and sausage. Worse, all these items served at an all-you-can-eat buffet.

➲ *Best opportunities:* Egg whites, orange and grapefruit juice, ham, oatmeal, whole-wheat bread with peanut butter and no-sugar-added preserves, fresh fruit (apples and bananas), lox (smoked salmon), protein bars and protein drinks.

Eating breakfast out can be a daily routine, something you do while traveling or part of business (meetings in restaurants or breakfast catered in the workplace). The restaurant industry has managed to fiercely maintain a meal rooted in agrarian culture—eggs from the henhouse, bacon from the pigs, butter from the cows, all fit for farmers working a vigorous sixteen-hour day. Oatmeal is offered in some sit-down restaurants, but it seems a poor-man's option when your colleagues are getting a full omelet with home fries and a side of pancakes.

Some health advisers suggest getting a toasted English muffin with fruit preserves when all else fails. I would be hungry within twenty minutes on a breakfast that small. Here are recommended strategies for negotiating the morning meal outside the home:

➲ *Quick morning stop:* Avoid fast food; go to a convenience store and get orange juice, a couple pieces of fruit, hard-boiled eggs, or beef jerky (yeah, beef jerky—it's a little high in sodium and therefore a bad idea for anyone with hypertension, but a one-ounce serving has about fifteen grams of protein and only half a gram of fat; just avoid brands that are high in nitrates, which are believed to be carcinogenic). Is there a health club on your route to work? Many serve protein drinks and other healthier foods such as whole-grain bagels with peanut butter, even to non-members; find out if you can phone your order in fifteen minutes before you get there (but check their nutrition facts for protein and sugar content).

➲ *Business meetings (in-office):* If it is politically feasible, talk to the human resources people or departmental administrative assistants to suggest getting away from Krispy Kremes and substituting salmon (lox), whole-grain bagels, fruit, and yogurt. It can make a world of difference to your health, but there is a business incentive as well: A better protein/carbohydrate balance will help workers maintain consistent energy levels (no high-carb sugar rush followed by a coma-inducing crash). If you are unsuccessful and stuck with donuts or Danishes, limit yourself to one, or avoid them altogether and grab a yogurt, protein drink, or protein bar beforehand.

➲ *Business meetings (restaurant):* A regular order of two scrambled eggs, four slices of bacon, and a serving of hash browns will give you 27 grams of protein and 43 grams of fat—far from your goal of a protein-to-fat ratio of 3:1. Many sit-down restaurants offer oatmeal, low-fat yogurt, fruit, and egg whites or egg substitutes.

## LUNCH

This lunch section presumes a casual meal, eaten solo or with colleagues. For more formal lunch meals, see the section on dinner.

➲ *Biggest pitfalls:* Fast-food cheeseburgers with fries; healthy-*sounding* sandwich fillers such as tuna, chicken, or turkey salad (all made with high-fat mayonnaise); skipping or skimping on lunch because you have to work through it, then getting bad vending-machine or snack-shop foods later in the afternoon. Or skipping lunch and an afternoon snack, leaving you completely ravenous and unable to make a reasonable decision about dinner.

➲ *Best opportunities:* Smart sandwiches; grab-and-go foods from convenience and grocery stores, including salad bars; health-Mex fajitas and burritos; green-leaf salads (in more of the major chains than ever before).

➲ *Fast-food options:* If you have few other choices, your best bets at the following major fast-food chains are detailed here. With a few exceptions, the recommended items are at or below fifteen grams of fat per serving. The "just for reference" selection shows how bad you can do when you're not paying attention. The absence of French fries in each is not an oversight; if you chronically consume fries, this is a great place to exercise your respect for vices. But if you gotta eat, you gotta eat—even when it's at a fast-food restaurant.

### McDonald's

*Chicken McGrill, no mayo:* 6 grams fat, 24 grams protein (300 calories). Mayo adds 11 grams fat and an additional 100 calories.

*Hamburger:* 10 grams fat, 12 grams protein (280 calories).

*Grilled Chicken Caesar Salad:* 7 grams fat, 26 grams protein (210 calories). Low-fat balsamic dressing adds 3 grams fat and no protein, and adds an additional 40 calories; other dressings are much higher in fat and calories.

*Fruit and Yogurt Parfait:* 4 grams fat, 8 grams protein (280 calories). Some McDonald's restaurants wisely serve this at breakfast, even though it is a dessert item.

JUST FOR REFERENCE . . .
Big Mac, Supersize Fries: 63 grams fat, 33 grams protein (1200 calories).

### Burger King
*Chicken Whopper with no mayo:* 9 grams fat, 38 grams protein (330 calories). Regular mayo adds 26 grams of fat and an additional 174 calories.
*Hamburger:* 13 grams fat, 17 grams protein (320 calories).
*Whopper, no mayo:* 28 grams fat, 34 grams protein (610 calories). Mayo adds 160 calories and 18 grams of fat.

JUST FOR REFERENCE . . .
Double Whopper with Cheese, King Fries: 106 grams fat, 71 grams protein (1720 calories).

### Wendy's
*Grilled Chicken Sandwich (no mayo):* 7 grams fat, 24 grams protein (300 calories).
*Chili, large:* 9 grams fat, 25 grams protein (300 calories).
*Spicy Chicken Sandwich (no mayo):* 15 grams fat, 27 grams protein (430 calories).
*Mandarin Chicken Salad with low-fat honey mustard dressing:* 18.5 grams fat, 25 grams protein (270 calories).

JUST FOR REFERENCE . . .
Big Bacon Classic, Biggie Fries: 52 grams fat, 30 grams protein (1100 calories).

### Taco Bell
In time, Taco Bell might start noticing the competition they are getting from upstart health-Mex chains (Chipotle Grill and others), and they'll use more black beans in place of the refried beans. Fat-free sour cream and maybe even grilled green peppers for fajitas would be good additions, too. In the meantime, a few items at least keep the fat level below fifteen grams per serving (Note: no item comes *close* to a 3:1 protein-to-fat ratio—and there are no *chalupas* in this list):

*Chicken Fiesta Burrito:* 12 grams fat, 17 grams protein (370 calories).
*Steak Fiesta Burrito:* 14 grams fat, 15 grams protein (370 calories).

*Bean Burrito:* 11 grams fat, 13 grams protein (370 calories).

*Chicken Soft Taco:* 7 grams fat, 13 grams protein (190 calories).

*Chicken Gordita Nacho Cheese:* 13 grams fat, 15 grams protein (290 calories).

*Steak Gordita Nacho:* 14 grams fat, 15 grams protein (290 calories).

JUST FOR REFERENCE . . .

Taco Salad with Salsa: 51 grams fat, 29 grams protein (850 calories). There are 30 grams of fat (and 5 grams of protein) in the shell alone, a clear case where the word "salad" does not connote "healthier."

### KFC

Roasted chicken offerings beat the fried chicken in all restaurants, but it's possible to lose half the fat from deep-fried fowl if you remove the skin. For a side, get the barbecue baked beans (1 gram fat, 8 grams protein).

*Drumstick:* 8 grams fat, 14 grams protein (140 calories).

*Whole Wing:* 9 grams fat, 11 grams protein (190 calories).

*Tender Roast Sandwich, no sauce:* 5 grams fat, 31 grams protein (270 calories). With sauce, add 14 grams fat and no additional protein (an additional 122 calories, or 392 calories total).

*Honey Barbecue–Flavored Sandwich:* 6 grams fat, 21 grams protein (300 calories).

JUST FOR REFERENCE . . .

Popcorn Chicken, large, and Potato Wedges: 56 grams fat, 33 grams protein (900 calories).

### Domino's Pizza

Although pizza is more traditionally considered a dinner food, many office lunch meetings are organized around this "Italian" favorite. Industry-wide pizza sales are annually around $30 billion, a number just about at a par with what we spend on burgers. At Domino's and other chains, and even mom-and-pop pizza parlors, a request can be made for half the normal amount of cheese, which will significantly increase the protein/fat ratio of your meal.

*Thin Crust Ham:* ¼ of a 12" pie (2 slices): 16.5 grams fat, 19 grams protein (375 calories).

*Thin Crust Cheese:* ¼ of a 12" pie (2 slices): 15.5 grams fat, 16.1 grams
protein (273 calories).

*Hand Tossed Veggie:* ¼ of a 12" pie (2 slices): 17 grams fat, 17 grams
protein (439 calories). Despite the cute and healthy *sounding* name,
it's higher in total calories than the one with ham. Blame the cheese.

JUST FOR REFERENCE . . .

Classic Hand Tossed ExtravaganZZa Feat Pizza (almost all the
ingredients they have back in the kitchen): ¼ of a 12" pie (2 slices): 27
grams fat, 27 grams protein (576 calories). If you eat the whole pie,
multiply these numbers by four.

# PROTEIN/FAT RATIO (PFR): YOUR PREFERENCE ON A MENU

**T**HE RELATIVE HEALTHFULNESS of a food item—how much
bang (favorable nutrients, such as protein) you get for your
buck—can be assessed according to its protein/fat ratio: the PFR or
"preference" measure. This is a simple, perhaps simplistic, means of
evaluating a restaurant menu item—simplistic because it doesn't take
into account other food values present in a meal (simple versus complex carbohydrates, fiber, and antioxidants). But looking at a menu
selection for its protein density, relative to fat, is a quick way to eval-
uate its relative healthfulness—a tool to help you keep within a protein-
leaning structure.

For example, a single (four-ounce) boneless/skinless breast of chicken
has about 30 grams of protein, less than 2 grams of fat, and no carbohydrates, and only about 160 calories. Stir-fried (restaurants say "sautéed")
with just a little olive oil, and some broccoli, tomatoes, and onions, chicken
gives you one very nutritious, high-protein/fat-ratio meal. Chicken coated in
breading and deep-fried (like "chicken tenders" or "chicken nuggets"),
served with fried onion rings and ketchup, has a lower PFR—the amount
of protein is constant while the fat portion is hiked up considerably.

Other examples:

**High PFR:**
■ Salmon sandwich on a whole-wheat roll with dark leafy greens,
garlic-fried green peppers (dense in omega-3 fatty acids, high-

quality protein, whole grains, vitamins, and minerals, including the antioxidants in garlic).

■ Roast beef with asparagus and sweet and sour cabbage soup (a lean meat, fibrous green vegetable, and nutrient-rich cabbage, low in fat, vitamins, and minerals).

■ Chicken burrito in the health-Mex version (whole beans, low-fat mozzarella, various vegetables; half or no white rice by request).

■ Egg-white omelet with low-fat mozzarella cheese, onions, tomatoes, hot sauce, whole-grain toast, and a side of berries (lean protein, lower-fat dairy with beneficial calcium, plant nutrients, whole-grain fiber, and vitamins and minerals).

**Low PFR:**

■ Burger with cheese and bacon, served on a white bun (saturated fats overwhelm the protein benefit, while the processed flour causes blood sugar to shoot up in a hurry).

■ Egg and sausage sandwich with hash browns (the whole-egg fat isn't the killer as much as the high-fat sausage and white-carb muffin that comes with it; add fried potatoes and butter and this meal should make you lethargic until lunchtime).

■ Pasta with cream sauce (white, not red) with seafood, chicken, or meat in sparse quantity (simple starches plus saturated fats that can slow you down for hours; minimal protein in the bits of fish, chicken, pork, or beef found in the sauce).

All foods and meals fall along a PFR continuum. You are going to benefit when you lean toward the high PFR side.

### Subway

Subway offers some of the best choices for easily maintaining a good protein/vegetable eating structure, especially when combined with lower-fat mayonnaise and salad dressing. The processed carbs are present in all choices of breads (even the wheat bread is not whole wheat), but that is mitigated by the fact that vegetables and lean meats are great choices. Choices listed below are all in half (six-inch) versions, but without cheese, dressing, and mayo. For a foot-long sandwich, double all values (note the difference in the meatball sub, below).

*Turkey Breast:* 3.5 grams fat, 16 grams protein (254 calories).
*Turkey Breast and Ham:* 4.5 grams fat, 18 grams protein (267 calories).
*Ham:* 4.5 grams fat, 17 grams protein (261 calories).
*Roast Beef:* 4.5 grams fat, 18 grams protein (264 calories).
*Roasted Chicken Breast:* 6 grams fat, 25 grams protein (311 calories).
*Veggie Delite (I hate the name, too):* 3 grams fat, 9 grams protein (200 calories).

JUST FOR REFERENCE . . .
Meatball *(foot-long):* 52 grams fat, 46 grams protein (1080 calories).

Note: All nutrition information was obtained from each restaurant chain's Web sites or in-store brochures. For links to more than seventy chain restaurants' nutritional data, go to www.nbez.info/restaur.shtml.

## DINNER

There are two ways to eat dinner out, each with a distinctly different dynamic: by yourself and with others. The nutrition challenges are similar, but you have more control when dining solo.

### Dinner on Your Own

➲ *Biggest pitfalls:* Restaurant owners make the best profits from alcohol sales, white carbohydrates (potatoes, breads, rice), and some lower-cost vegetables. The baskets of bread on the table may be free, but, except in the rare instances when it is made from whole grains, the virtually unlimited supply of rolls, French baguettes, and Italian bread costs a lot in our healthy-eating plan (each slice of Italian or French bread has about eighty calories and one gram of fat).

➲ *Best opportunities:* Eat the healthy foods that are most difficult for you to make at home. Fish is on more menus than ever before, while the leaner roast beef and steaks can be healthful options. There's always the chicken, and you can practice your skills at vice management by setting a limit on how much of that free bread you absolutely need to consume.

# ANOTHER GOOD REASON TO GET THE SALMON OR TROUT

**Y**OU MIGHT AVOID FISH, perhaps because of some bad childhood experience. In my case, it was going to the Rockland (Maine) Lobster Festival at the age of five and being fed weird white crustacean stuff when I'd rather have had a hamburger. But for the sake of better health, maybe you can give *pesce* a chance, at least once a month.

According to a report published in the *Journal of the American Medical Association* (December 2002), Dr. Ka He and collaborators at Harvard's School of Public Health found that men who ate about three to five ounces of fish just one to three times a month were 43 percent less likely to have a stroke during twelve years of follow-up. Men who ate fish more often did not reduce their risk any further, suggesting that a small amount of fish works just as well as a larger one (as it affects stroke incidence—other health benefits come from more frequent fish meals). Why? Researchers say it probably has something to do with omega-3 fatty acids, which lower the levels of blood fats that are linked to cardiovascular disease and which help prevent unwanted blood clotting. Fish highest in omega-3s are (in descending order) salmon, trout, herring, swordfish, oysters, and pollock. Canned tuna contains some omega-3s, but in only $\frac{1}{15}$th the concentration of that of salmon; shrimp and crab have slightly more than tuna; and lobster ranks lowest, with $\frac{1}{30}$th the concentration of omega-3s found in salmon.

If you don't feel like making it yourself, a restaurant is the best place to get fish. Try ordering fish the first time it's offered to you after the first of each month. Be sure to get it broiled, baked, blackened, grilled, or steamed—*not* fried, stuffed, or with cream, cheese, butter, tartar sauce, or a cracker crust.

If you are traveling and eating off a hotel room-service menu, you obviously are not bargain hunting. So choosing a healthy menu option is not a cost consideration. If there is no reasonably healthy offering on the menu, inquire at the front desk or concierge about ordering in from neighborhood restaurants. At a minimum, you'll get broader choices.

### Dinner with Others

➲ *Biggest pitfalls:* Exacerbating the pitfalls mentioned above, you have the added difficulty of choosing a restaurant among compatriots with different agendas. If attempts to influence colleagues to select a healthier establishment fail, buck up and work your way through the menu to find fruits and vegetables, lean meats, complex carbohydrates, and lower-fat dairy products where you can.

➲ *Best opportunities:* Sometimes being forced to try new restaurants exposes you to new healthful foods. Look for different types of vegetables, spices, and other flavors and unusual combinations—for example, raspberries with balsamic vinegar—to broaden your own cooking skills.

Meat, pork, fish, or fowl—all animal proteins—are usually the centerpiece of the meal eaten in most types of restaurants. Because it's impractical to recommend specific items to order, your best tactic is to become familiar with how different cuts and preparation methods rank in general protein density. The best choices for ethnic restaurants follow.

## PROTEIN/FAT RATIO (PFR) MENU GUIDE

THIS GUIDE SHOULD ASSIST you in ordering a leaner protein source when eating out. The list is ordered by animal type and cuts in **ascending order of fat and calorie content.** As selections get denser in fat and calories, the **PFR** (as defined here by proportion of protein to fat and calorie content of an item) **declines.** In other words, the items listed first are preferable to those that follow. This assumes a consistent use of the healthiest preparation methods (broiling or grilling, not frying) unless specifically indicated, and none of these foods should be served in butter or cream sauces. PFRs of items sharing a line are roughly equivalent.

1. Cod, crab, monkfish, octopus, pike, pollock, scallops, scrod, skate
2. Striped bass, mussels, northern lobster, oysters, perch, red snapper, sea bass, squid (most often served as calamari), turbot
3. Abalone, halibut, king mackerel, sea trout, shrimp, smelt, yellowfin and skipjack tuna

4. Freshwater bass, bluefish, catfish, mullet, sturgeon, swordfish, rainbow trout, salmon (chum and pink)
5. Turkey (white meat, no skin)
6. Lamb (chops and leg of lamb)
7. Chicken (breast, no skin)
8. Carp, orange roughy, whitefish, shark
9. Turkey (dark meat, no skin)
10. Milkfish, salmon (coho and Atlantic), other varieties of trout, bluefish tuna, yellowtail
11. Beef: Sirloin steak, New York, club, delmonico, strip steak, filet mignon, filet steak, medallions, London broil, kabob, roast beef, pot roast, stew and soup meat, stir-fry meat; pork: ham, pork tenderloin
12. Atlantic herring, other mackerel, haddock
13. Pheasant (with skin), turkey (white meat, with skin), chicken (white meat, with skin and dark meat, no skin), duck (no skin)
14. Chinook and sockeye salmon, fish cakes (fried), squid (fried)
15. Chicken (dark meat, with skin), turkey (dark meat, with skin), goose (no skin), chicken (white meat and "fingers," fried)
16. Veal (roast, fat trimmed), London broil (fat on*), roast beef (fat on), kabobs (fat on)
17. Fat-trimmed** beef: prime rib, rib steak, rib eye steak, brisket, corned beef, beef fajitas, ribs, porterhouse, T-bone
18. Fat-trimmed pork: Pork loin, pork chop
19. Shad, sablefish, Geenland halibut
20. Chicken (dark meat, fried)
21. Sirloin steak (fat on), beef short ribs (fat trimmed), pork ribs (fat trimmed), beef and pork tongue
22. Fried (all): scallops, catfish, red snapper, shrimp
23. Fat-on beef: Porterhouse steak, T-bone, prime rib, filet mignon, "chicken fried" steak, beef chitterlings; fat-on pork: pork loin, tenderloin
24. Goose (skin on)
25. Beef and pork sausage
26. Fat-on beef ribs, meatloaf, lamb chops, pork chops, pork ribs, spareribs
27. Chicken wings (fried), duck with skin
28. Bass (stuffed and baked), eel (fried), mackerel (fried), smelt (fried)

**29.** Beef brisket (fat on)

**30.** Short ribs (fat on)

*Also described as "untrimmed"

**Must be specified on the menu or by wait staff as "trimmed," as all cuts come in untrimmed versions as well.

> Source: Derived from *Dining Lean: How to Eat Healthy in Your Favorite Restaurants (Without Feeling Deprived)*, Joanne V. Lichten, R.D., Ph.D., Nutrifit Publishing, 2000.

Scan this list and you'll see that grilled pork tenderloin beats out fried chicken—happy news to red-meat carnivores. But take into account what comes with all items (German-style coleslaw or mashed potatoes?); be assertive about asking for substitutes if they don't offer a smart combination.

One important caveat: "Leaner" isn't the only indicator of a "healthy" meal. Variety counts—you're more likely to appreciate seafood (over short ribs) if you order a different fish every time. But fish high in omega-3 fatty acids—salmon, trout, herring, and others—are lower on the list because it's their fat that carries the goods. Also, a rib eye steak served with fresh greens and a black bean soup would be a meal high in fiber, protein, and iron, and great to order once in a while. Balance, variety, and moderation are your ultimate keys.

## GOING ETHNIC

IN OUR GREAT MULTICULTURAL society, foods of the world have come to almost every city in North America. In fact, I'm often amazed to think how some families born on the other side of the earth picked up and moved kids and kettles to some midwestern town they couldn't possibly have dreamed of while watching reruns of *Dynasty* dubbed into Mandarin or Hindi. And we get to eat the interesting and sometimes healthy foods that they brought with them.

Except America has a way of changing some things. To appeal to our tastes, many ethnic foods are altered with more meat, more cheese, fewer vegetables, or more fat. For example, quick-serve Chinese food found in shopping-mall food courts is as far from the native form as Boston is from Beijing. But not to panic, many great and healthy foods can be found. Here are things to look for when eating international:

# ASIAN FOODS
# (CHINESE, JAPANESE AND SUSHI, THAI, VIETNAMESE)

Episodes of *South Park* featuring the restaurant City Wok (Cartman and pals like to phone the owner just to hear him mispronounce the name) bear testimony to the extent the Far East has invaded the Western world with moderately priced, *potentially* healthy food. And we like it. But there's great variance between foods of these different cultures, and even within them, when it comes to maintaining a smart eating structure. Like most restaurant foods, Asian food tends to be high in sodium. Some tips on what to order:

### Chinese

Chinese menus are known for providing many choices. Look for:

⊃ Hot and sour soup: tasty use of spices, meat, and tofu, fairly low in fat
⊃ Szechwan shrimp: pairs low-fat shrimp with stir-fried vegetables
⊃ Most things with tofu—the protein product of soybeans commonly used in Asian cooking—as long as they are not *deep*-fried (*stir*-fried is OK)
⊃ Steamed dumplings in place of the fried version, with either shrimp or vegetables (also avoid fried egg rolls and fried spring rolls)
⊃ Chop Suey, a mix of meat and vegetables, but not chow mein, which usually has fried noodles on top
⊃ Chicken and broccoli, not deep-fried
⊃ Lemon chicken, not deep-fried
⊃ Chicken in garlic sauce, not deep-fried
⊃ Steamed vegetables and chicken, shrimp, or tofu

But watch out for:

⊃ Fast-food Chinese: See how the meat glistens in the light? To speed the cooking process once your order is placed, they often pre-cook the meat in a deep fryer, then hold it for the lunch or dinner hour, when they stir-fry it—the meat is fried twice. Dim sum, poo poo platter, lobster sauce, Peking duck, spareribs, Cantonese sauces, egg rolls, and spring rolls—all bad.

### Japanese and Sushi

Sushi is one of the most popular and healthy foods to emerge from the Land of the Rising Sun. In Japan, it's served as an appetizer or side dish. Here, we have turned it into an expensive, full-course meal. Even without the sake, you can easily spend $50 wolfing down these dainty bites of uncooked fish (wolfing is not so common in most Honshu prefectures). But talk about tasty—the ginger and wasabi (green stuff) make my mouth tingle.

Elsewhere on a full Japanese restaurant menu, things get a little dicey. "Tempura" is coated and deep-fried vegetables (or other foods such as shrimp), something you'd expect to emerge from American corporate food development. But there are still great, close-to-the-farm dishes in more traditional Japanese restaurants. Look for:

- ➲ Miso soup (soy and spinach or seaweed), as well as suimono, su-udon and yaki-udon (all soups)
- ➲ Green salad (with ginger dressing)
- ➲ Fish (most kinds)
- ➲ Teriyaki chicken or shrimp
- ➲ Sushi and sashimi
- ➲ Edamame (soybeans in the pod)
- ➲ Steamed dumplings

### Thai

I consider Thai, along with Vietnamese and Mongolian, to be the healthiest and tastiest bet when it comes to Asian food. Thai restaurants serve foods steamed, boiled, or roasted more often than fried, and with fresh cilantro, other herbs, nuts, and chilis that are both strong and satisfying tastes. The abundance of plants used in their foods is attributable to the fact that Thailand is located in a monsoon region with rich soil. Look for:

- ➲ Fresh spring rolls with chicken, vegetables, and/or shrimp (steamed, not fried)

➲ Satay (chicken and peanut butter sauce, but try to leave some of the sauce on the plate—it could cause you to exceed your weekly quota of peanut butter)
➲ Wing bean salad (tom kha kai)
➲ Soups: hot shrimp, tom yum goong, talay thong
➲ Swamp-cabbage hot salad (don't knock it till you've tried it)
➲ Green hot curry with chicken, but not if it has coconut milk
➲ Sweet-and-sour pork

. . . and many other main dishes featuring lean meats with generous portions of vegetables

But watch out for:

➲ Anything deep-fried (again, largely a concession to American tastes)
➲ Carb-heavy white rice and, I'm sad to acknowledge, delicious pad Thai (get it once in a while if you really like it)

### Vietnamese

Nutritionally similar to Thai food, Vietnamese restaurants have grown exponentially in the Americas since the fall of Saigon. There are broad variations from restaurant to restaurant on which foods are used and how they are made and named, so a specific list of what to order here is elusive. Stick to your smart-eating structure (lean meats and vegetables, not fried), and notice the two or three fresh herbs with each dish. Take some ideas home with you.

## CAJUN/CREOLE

The twists of history and migrations took food-loving French and other European peoples to the seafood- and spice-rich regions of the Gulf of Mexico and the Caribbean, and ultra-spicy and blackened foods resulted. We now associate them with festive times (Mardi Gras and other drinking occasions in general); guys are among the cuisine's biggest fans.

The seafood is a step in the right direction, but about half the dishes are fried. Finding your way through a Cajun (based in Louisiana) or Creole (based in Caribbean, Central American, and some American Gulf states) shouldn't be too difficult if you avoid the fried food.

➲ Choose red (cocktail) sauces over tartar or butter to save significantly on fat.

➲ Look out for "stuffed" anything. It's usually breaded and full of oil.

➲ Red beans and rice are made to order for your eating plan (pick through the rice to get more of the beans).

## INDIAN/PAKISTANI

Immigrants from the Indian subcontinent have done a fine job of introducing us to tandoori chicken and scads of dishes made with curry. It's an amazingly rich culture with both healthy and too-rich foods—Ghandi was thin because he went on hunger strikes, not as a result of a vegetarian diet (India's Buddhists are vegetarian, the Muslims don't eat pork, and the Hindus don't eat beef, so this may not be the best choice of cuisine for avid carnivores). Restaurants combine flavors and dishes from widely disparate provinces.

Look for:

➲ Soups with lentils and vegetables
➲ Main and side dishes incorporating garbanzos (e.g., aloo chole)
➲ Chicken and fish dishes (tandoori, tikka, vindaloo, and masala)
➲ Kabobs of chicken, shrimp, and lamb
➲ Chutney, a mix of chopped fruit, onions, and spices

But watch out for:

➲ Anything made with coconut milk (tropical oils from coconuts and palm are highly saturated)
➲ Fried bread (paratha)
➲ Other fried appetizers (papadum, samosas, and pakoras)

## ITALIAN

So mainstream this may not need its own ethnic category, Italian food got a great surge of popularity in the "carb-up" 1980s. Even in the low-fat 90s, we felt good about a big plate of pasta topped with red sauce. Italians use a lot of those great lycopene-rich tomatoes, plus tons of eggplants, peppers, fresh basil, oregano, lemon, and olive oil. But the amount of refined carbohydrates in the pasta—served in portions that might have fed an entire family in Calabria during the Mussolini era—push this food into high-carb territory (desirable whole-wheat, spinach, and soy-based pastas are more available than before, but are still rare in Italian restaurants).

Order your appetizer and main dish with lean meat in mind, and in particular look for the following:

➲ Seafood (squid, mussels, clams, and fish with fins), in a red (marinara) or light wine sauce (piccata or marsala), broiled, not fried or in a butter or cream sauce.
➲ Bean (*fagioli*) and minestrone soups (high in protein)
➲ Salads in vinaigrette dressing
➲ Chicken or veal cacciatore

But watch out for:

➲ Lasagna (largely refined grain pasta, loaded with saturated fat from cheese)
➲ Eggplant and chicken parmigiana (excessive cheese and oil)
➲ Fettucine alfredo (to your stomach, it's just another form of macaroni and cheese)
➲ Baked ziti (like lasagna, mostly a meal of processed carbs and saturated cheese fat)

## MEXICAN

There are three kinds of Mexican foods available north of the border. They are fast food (major chains and independents, including the newer health-Mex style), Margaritavilles (sit down, drink until you are seeing double, then eat a meal you'll never remember), and finer cuisine (upscale restaurants that present a whole different, and healthier, type of meal, using fish, plant foods, and often citrus). Because the fast-food versions are discussed elsewhere in this chapter, the advice provided here is more applicable to the latter two types. It's tricky territory. Some tips:

➲ Chips and salsa: Salsa could hardly be a richer source of healthy vegetables, herbs, and spices. The chips, on the other hand, are processed carbohydrates and fat (about one gram of fat per chip). Some restaurants offer them baked instead of fried, which is a small step in the right direction. Put either type in front of me and I usually eat the whole basket. Then I ask for a second. My strategy is to scoop up a lot of salsa on one chip, then eat it slowly. I still end up eating a lot, but I eat more salsa in balance with the chips. A smarter approach is to ask the waiter to take them away, but dinner companions are unlikely to settle for that. This is a dilemma with no easy answer for guys with appetites. Maybe you can think about how too many chips will slow down absorption of your margaritas?

➲ Refried beans have twice the processing and four times the fat of whole beans. Avoid.

➲ Chicken fajitas: In a corn (not flour) tortilla (not taco shell), this is one of your best bets, giving you a lean meat with vegetables (usually onions and green peppers). Back off on the sour cream if you can, but guacamole, fatty as it is, has good, plant-based unsaturated fat.

➲ Chicken enchiladas: As with fajitas, hold off on the sour cream and scoop off the cheese on top. Otherwise, it's good lean meat with a tomato-based sauce.

➲ Camarones de haca: Shrimp in a tomato or tomatillo sauce, this can be a winner.

➲ Arroz con pollo: Arroz (rice) might be a little too carb-heavy, but served with enough pollo (chicken) you at least are getting a good dose of lean meat. Get a side of salsa and bean soup and you're in business.

➲ Ceviche is a good bet.

➲ Gazpacho is a healthy soup.

➲ Soft chicken or seafood tacos are fine if you lay off the sour cream.

➲ Tamales are also a healthy choice.

## NORTH AFRICAN (ALGERIAN, MOROCCAN, AND TUNISIAN)

This region of Africa on the Mediterranean coast was a trade crossroads for centuries, endowing the cultures with spices, and vegetables that seem remarkably American (celery, beans, carrots, tomatoes, potatoes, spinach, and cauliflower). But what's most appealing to the provincial North American guy might be the fact that about one-third of the plate in North African eating establishments is covered with beef, poultry, lamb, or fish. The spices they favor are fairly familiar—black pepper, paprika, chili, caraway, fennel, saffron, cinnamon, and cumin—but it's the amount they use that might blow you away. The Tunisians tend to favor hot and red spices, Moroccans lean toward the yellowish saffron (especially in the rice), and the Algerians strike a balance between the two. Go easy on the flat breads, but don't hesitate to try their many stews—they are meaty, hearty, and very tasty.

Look for:

⊃ Lamb, fish, chicken, or beef on kababs
⊃ Dishes containing almonds and pecans
⊃ Hummus, baba ghanoush, and dolma (stuffed grape leaves)— also staples of Middle Eastern and Greek food, they contain oil, mashed garbanzo beans, and great plant foods (parsley, leafy vegetables). All good stuff.

But watch out for:

⊃ Potato-heavy dishes
⊃ Rice-heavy dishes (unless they serve wild rice—higher-priced restaurants tend to do that more often)
⊃ Fried versions of foods like squid (calamari) and falafel (not exactly North African foods, but frequently served in American North African restaurants).

## MIDDLE EASTERN

These are the foods that come from the eastern end of the Mediterranean, including Greece, Lebanon, Turkey, Armenia, Syria, Iran, and Iraq. Due to heavy use of plant foods (garbanzo beans, eggplant, cracked wheat, lentils, olives, tomatoes, herbs, and spices) with relatively little processing, Middle Eastern foods can be quite healthy. Note that Arabic physicians in the Middle Ages used diets rich in plant foods as medicine; European soldiers in the Crusades took the technique back to their homelands.

Things to look for:

⊃ Baba ghanoush (eggplant mixed with Tahini and spices)
⊃ Chicken in pita break (pockets)
⊃ Hummus (mashed garbanzos with olive oil, lemon juice, and tahini—sometimes without oil)
⊃ Kafta (grilled beef with spices)

➲ Kibbeh (cracked wheat, meat, sautéed onions, and pine nuts)
➲ Lentil soup (a high-protein legume served with vegetables)
➲ Shish kababs (grilled meat and vegetables)
➲ Souvlaki (marinated and grilled fish and chicken)
➲ Tabouli (cracked wheat with parsley, tomatoes, and spices)

But watch out for:

➲ Spanakopita
➲ Phyllo dough
➲ Cavia
➲ Bibbeh

. . . all nutritionally inferior because of processed grains and fats (oil or lard).

## CHALLENGING OCCASIONS

LIFE SOMETIMES HANDS US limited choices, even when our hunger is most pronounced. Having a strategy for such times is essential, particularly when you know that such events—post-workout, while traveling, and during social events and working meals—can be frequent. For the smart-eating guy, every problem has a solution.

### THE GYM, POST-WORKOUT

For guys who work out, this is a distinct part of the day. Morning and lunchtime workouts should be immediately followed by a meal, but with evening exercise eating is trickier because of the need to go to bed soon afterward.

➲ *Biggest pitfalls:* After a workout, particularly in the evening, one school of thought might be "I've just exercised so I can eat what I want." But a few greasy burgers and fries can pretty well wipe out any gains at the gym. Also, many gyms offer fruit smoothies and other foods that are inappropriately high in simple sugars (check the basic ingredients if you can; clubs with a staff dietitian are most reliable).

⊃ *Best opportunities:* Protein bars and drinks (along with multiple other supplements) can be made with real fruit and a good proportion of whey protein. If your club offers nutrition counseling, by all means meet with the registered dietitian or another credentialed nutritionist to learn more about specific dietary recommendations following a workout. Most dietitians encourage consumption of readily digested protein (along with a moderate amount of carbohydrates) within an hour following strength training or other rigorous exercise to help build and repair muscle tissue. In general, however, a balanced meal (of fruits, vegetables, lean meats, low-fat dairy, and complex carbohydrates, available in some clubs) will best serve your overall physiological needs. Also keep in mind that a good night's sleep is an essential component of muscle development, so a simple, small, and quick meal can help you hit the hay sooner.

## TRAVEL

Because travel (and its disruption of eating and overall health) is so prevalent in modern life, here is a special section organized by various modes of transport.

### Airports and Airplanes

⊃ *Biggest pitfalls:* You eat what they put in front of you because your next-best options are thirty thousand feet or several hours away. And while the trend is for airports to offer more food courts and restaurants, have you ever been stranded in an airport with minimal eating options, particularly during late-night hours? A vending machine might be your only choice.

⊃ *Best opportunities:* Some airlines offer in-flight healthy eating options, while airport restaurants are increasing their healthful meal choices as well (see table on page 267). With the growth of no-meal flights, you do not appear quite so odd if you bring your own food on board.

### Rules of Thumb for Eating When Flying

Your first smart move is to eat well before leaving home, but for extended travel (flights lasting three or more hours), supplement the carrier's food with your own smart snacks (protein bars, carrots, hummus, apples, peanut butter, low-fat cheese, yogurt, etc.).

Many carriers offer special meals (diabetic, cardiac or heart-healthy, vegetarian, kosher, Hindu, reduced sodium, etc.). However, not all of these meals are necessarily lower in fat and higher in protein than the regular meal. Your best bet would be to go for the cardiac meal—it is at least lower in fat and sodium.

The following breakdown of offerings on major carriers, assessed by Nutricize.com, provides a glimpse of how challenging it can be to maintain a good eating structure during a flight.

**AIRLINE MEALS—OVERVIEW OF NUTRITIONAL VALUE**

*Sample Dinner—Coach Class*

| Airline | Calories | Protein (g) | Fat (g) |
|---|---|---|---|
| American | 824 | 47 | 50 |
| America West | 847 | 25 | 32 |
| Continental | 1,304 | 43 | 76 |
| Northwest | 854 | 37 | 37 |
| Qantas | 1,164 | 44 | 62 |
| TWA | 1,019 | 33 | 59 |
| **United** | **723** | **39** | **13** |
| US Airways | 1,022 | 63 | 54 |
| **Midwest Airlines** | **1,643** | **53** | **91** |
| Lufthansa | 1,419 | 47 | 83 |
| JAL | 1,219 | 58 | 51 |
| Delta | 1,104 | 57 | 54 |
| **British Airways** | **534** | **28** | **21** |
| Virgin Atlantic | 1,168 | 36 | 53 |
| Air France | 959 | 58 | 43 |
| **AVERAGE** | **1,054** | **45** | **52** |

United is highlighted because its menu alone offers a meal with a protein-to-fat ratio of 3:1, our target proportion. British Airways wins in the calorie department, but has a poor protein-to-fat ratio. Midwest Airlines ranks at the bottom in all respects. The numbers in this table indicate a general disregard for nutrition on the part of the airlines; responsibility for smart eating falls on you.

# "YOUR FLIGHT HAS BEEN DELAYED"

**A** STORM IN DENVER MIGHT divert your flight to Chicago, which makes your life—and your meals—take on a whole different schedule. A couple of days in the same clothes might be bad enough; you should at least try not to eat popcorn for breakfast. A survey of airport restaurants by the Physicians Committee for Responsible Medicine, a nonprofit health organization that promotes preventive health measures, including good nutrition, identified information about airports around the country. Following is a list of airports, the number of healthy restaurants out of the total number of restaurants in each airport, and the percentage of healthy restaurants:

> San Francisco Airport (SFO): 24 out of 25; 96 percent
> Minneapolis–St. Paul Airport (MSP): 27 out of 41; 66 percent
> Chicago–O'Hare Airport (ORD): 18 out of 28; 64 percent
> Denver Airport (DEN): 14 out of 23; 61 percent
> Los Angeles Airport (LAX): 21 out of 35; 60 percent
> Phoenix Airport (PHX): 25 out of 43; 58 percent
> Dallas–Fort Worth Airport (DFW): 28 out of 56; 50 percent
> Las Vegas Airport (LAS): 13 out of 29; 45 percent
> Atlanta Airport (ATL): 17 out of 42; 40 percent
> Detroit Metro Airport (DTW): 9 out of 27; 33 percent

Note: Restaurants rated "healthy" offered at least one low-fat, high-fiber, cholesterol-free entrée.

Source: PCRM's "Airport Food Ratings 2001: Availability of Healthy Food Choices, the Ten Busiest Airports in the Country, from Best to Worst."

### Highways

○ *Biggest pitfalls:* You are a captive of the interstate highway system and the handful of national fast-food retailers and truck-stop diners that cluster around exits. Your two main dietary interests could well be caffeine to stay alert and processed carbohydrates to ease the stomach discomfort from too much coffee.

○ *Best opportunities:* Pack a cooler with your own healthier snacks: bags of baby carrots, fruit and fruit juices, water, nuts, peanut butter, hard-boiled eggs, whole-wheat pretzels with mustard, and sandwiches, such as peanut butter on whole wheat, hummus with lettuce and tomato and cucumbers). When that runs out, practice smart eating habits as you would on any fast-food and restaurant occasion. Part of being alert is having moderate levels of sugar and insulin in your bloodstream (which donuts, French fries, and other processed foods will not accomplish).

### Extended Stays on the Road

➲ *Biggest pitfalls:* Lacking cooking facilities, awareness of area restaurants, and time, it is easy to default to either room service and its limitations, or fast-food joints that are open when you need to eat and predictable.

➲ *Best opportunities:* If you plan to be in the same hotel (or the home of friends who don't keep smart food stocked in their houses) for three or more days, look for the closest grocery or convenience store to stock up on apples, bananas, dried fruit, and nuts. If your hotel has a coffeemaker, you can use it to boil water to make oatmeal. If it has a microwave and mini-refrigerator, get orange juice, egg substitutes, and yogurt for mornings and snacks. You might even buy canned beans and frozen chicken entrées.

## BUSINESS-MEETING MEALS

➲ *Biggest pitfalls:* Because business meals are organized to either keep the troops working through the meal or to generate camaraderie, nutrition often takes a backseat to these other concerns. To eat light or get your meal elsewhere might even be considered bad form in many companies. Another inexplicable custom is the mid-afternoon cookie meetings. If you weren't falling asleep yet, those oatmeal or chocolate chip confections can work like sleeping pills. Avoid them. Have a protein bar, peanuts, or an apple on hand as your afternoon snack.

➲ *Best opportunities:* Get involved in the planning process, if possible, to introduce your colleagues to the benefits of increased productivity from healthier eating. Show engagement and strategic thinking by gathering menus from area restaurants that can cater such meals. If the "meal" is merely snacks of donuts, Danishes, cookies, or chips, you are not obligated to partake.

## DINNER PARTIES AND COCKTAIL BUFFETS

⊃ *Biggest pitfalls:* Because someone went to a lot of trouble and expense to provide you with exotic and indulgent foods, you feel obligated to eat lots of everything (if you're like my frugal Uncle Harvey, you skip a meal or two before going just to take full advantage). Also, when alcohol and a general sense of conviviality are present, smart eating disappears.

⊃ *Best opportunities:* Enjoy yourself and let your hosts know how much you appreciate their hospitality. They won't notice when you eat only a tiny or single portion of everything. Look for their own creative use of smart foods (fruits and vegetables, lean meats, low-fat dairy, and whole grains) and compliment them by asking how they were prepared; then see if you can replicate such dishes on your own. And if experience tells you that a particular host makes everything in a deep-fryer, bring your own contribution of a bean salad or something else to the event. The host will think that you are the most generous guest, when in fact you are just ensuring that you have something suitable to eat.

## NEXT TIME THE SMELL OF BUTTERED POPCORN WAFTS INTO THE ROOM

Regardless of the time and place, food confronts you at almost every waking moment. Your instincts tell you to eat everything in sight as soon as possible. But the physiological feast/famine triggers do not serve modern needs, so you need to remember the following:

⊃ **Stick with your at-home habits.** Keep your smart-eating structure in your head at all times. At each time when a decision is to be made (where to eat and what to order), remember that you *prefer* fruits and vegetables, lean meat, whole grains, and low-fat dairy, prepared and served in a way closest to nature. For example, grilled beef (or chicken or fish) and vegetables, not battered and fried meat, or anything rolled up into a pastry shell.

⊃ **Snack.** For solo meals on the go, eat one thing to tide you over until later (e.g., a small bag of nuts). Or if persuaded by others to go to a restaurant with few (or no) good options, eat some apples or carrots beforehand just to reduce space in your stomach for the bad stuff to come. There's almost always a chicken sandwich on the menu; just skip the fries and get a vegetable as a substitute.

⊃ **Be persuasive.** For group meals, be willing to assert your interest in a healthier restaurant. Don't be a jerk about it, but at least state your interest so friends and colleagues give it some thought ("Gee, we go there a lot. Why not try that new health-Mex place?"). Chances are that several others will agree with you and follow your lead.

⊃ **Think and act "big picture."** If all else fails and you find yourself eating fried onion loaf while waiting for the triple-decker cheeseburger, resolve that over the next two or three days you are going to eat a lot of vegetables and fruit. Maybe even save room for a grapefruit dessert when you get home (after a salty meal, at the very least you'll need the water found in citrus).

You will not always be successful. Eating out, like life itself, usually involves some compromise. But you probably will make an improvement when you dine with your smart-eating plan in mind—and you'll achieve balance, variety, and moderation.

You gotta eat. Discover how great it can be when you do it smart.

# bibliography

Agatston, Arthur. *The South Beach Diet*. Emmaus, PA: Rodale Press, 2003.

Ash, Russell. *The Top 10 of Everything 2002*. New York: DK Publishing, 2001.

Atkins, Robert C. *Dr. Atkins' New Diet Revolution*. New York: Avon/HarperCollins, 2001.

Bartoshuk, Linda. (Yale University School of Medicine. linda.bartoshuk@yale.edu) Ability to taste is sex related (Book on nutrition for men) [Internet]. Message to: Russ Klettke (KlettkeRus@aol .com), 2002 November 25, 2:49 p.m. [11 lines].

Boyles, Salynn. Atkins Diet Works; Safety Unknown. WebMD Medical News reviewed by Michael Smith, M.D. [Internet] 2002, July 18. Available from: http://aolsvc.health.webmd.aol.com/ content/article/49/39679.htm

Brand-Miller, Jennie, et al. *The Glucose Revolution*. New York: Marlowe & Company, 1999.

Brand-Miller, Jennie, et al. *The Glucose Revolution Life Plan*. New York: Marlowe & Company, 2001.

Candel, M. J. J. M. "Consumers' convenience orientation towards meal preparation: conceptualization and measurement." *Appetite* 36, no. 1 (2001): 15–28.

Castleman, Michael. *The New Healing Herbs*. Emmaus, PA: Rodale Press, 2001.

Centers for Disease Control, National Center for Chronic Disease Prevention and Health Promotion. Obesity Trends, prevalence of obesity among U.S. Adults, Region and State. [Internet]. 2002 May 13. Available from: http://www.ded.gov/nccdphp/dnpa/obesity/trend/prev_reg.htm

Editors, *Men's Health* magazine. *The* Men's Health *Belly-Off Program*. Emmaus, PA: Rodale Press, 2002.

Elliot, Rose. *Vegetarian Fast Food*. New York: Random House, 1994.

Evans, William, and Irwin H. Rosenberg. *Biomarkers: The Ten Keys to Prolonging Vitality*. New York: Simon & Schuster/Fireside, 1991.

Fox, Maggie. Supersize portions cause obesity. Reuters News Service, 2002 October 24.

Falcon, Mike, and Stephen Shoop. SuperBowl ads neglect nutrition. *USA Today*, 2001 January 29.

Fast Food's Most Decadent Burger Arrives at Jack in the Box® Restaurants [Internet]. [Cited: 2001 April 13]: Available from: http://www.jackinthebox.com/pressroom/pressreleases/pr.php?UID =17&Year=2001

Fitzgerald, Matt. The benefits of eating whole foods; Lose fat and live longer by getting back to basic foods. *Men's Fitness* online [Internet]. 2002 July 22: Available from: http://rx.fitnessonline.com/content/6205.jsp.

Fox, Maggie. Tea may reduce risk of cancer, heart disease. Reuters News Agency, 2002 September 24.

Gittleman, Ann Louise. *Super Nutrition for Men*. New York: Avery Publishing Group, 1999.

Goldberg, Kenneth, et al. *The Men's Health Longevity Program*. Emmaus, PA: Rodale Press, 2001.

Grocery Manufacturers of America. Opinion '98: Marketplace trends in grocery shopping [Internet]: Available from: http://www.gmabrands.com/facts/opinion98/04.cfm.

Hellmich, Nanci. College eating habits are clogged with fat. *USA Today*, 2002 January 10.

Hellmich, Nanci. Those big portions are getting even bigger. *USA Today*, 2002 March 3.

International Health, Racquet & Sportsclub Association. "Industry fares well in 2001." IHRSA Trend Report: Economic Outlook for 2002: 9, no. 1.

Information Resources, Inc. Snack Foods' Popularity Increases. *Supermarket News*, 2001 May 7.

Jacobson, Michael F., et al. *Restaurant Confidential*. New York: Workman Publishing, 2002.

Klein, Barbara. Nutrient conservation in canned, frozen and fresh foods. Urbana-Champaign, IL, University of Illinois, Department of Food Science and Human Nutrition: 1997 October .

Kunz, Gray, and Peter Kaminsky. *The Elements of Taste*. New York: Little Brown & Company, 2001.

Lichten, Joanne. *Dining Lean: How to Eat Healthy in Your Favorite Restaurants*. Houston: Nutrifit Publishing, 1998.

Lucier, Gary. French Fry Markets Continue to Sizzle. *Agricultural Outlook* [Internet]. 1996 October: Available from: http://www.fas .usda.gov/htp2/circular/1996/96-10/oct96htp1.html.

Magee, Elaine. *Taste vs. Fat*. Minneapolis: Chronimed Publishing (John Wiley & Sons, NY), 1997.

Mann, Bill. Calling all male shoppers. San Francisco: CBS Marketwatch [Internet].1999 October 21: Available from: http://americasresearchgroup.com/male_shoppers.html.

Media Department, Food Marketing Institute. Consumers Cite Value and Nutrition as Primary Drivers for Shopping Decisions, According to FMI's Trends 2002. Chicago: 2002 May 7.

Mokdad, A. H., M. Serdula, et al. "The spread of the obesity epidemic in the United States, 1991–1998." *Journal of the American Medical Association* 282 (1999): 1519–22.

Mokdad A.H., et al. "The continuing epidemics of obesity and diabetes in the United States." *Journal of the American Medical Association* 286 (2001): 1195–1200).

Moore, John Frederick. E-Business Dispatch [Internet]. Why Peapod is thriving: first-failure advantage. Available from: http://business2 .com/search?qt=peapod+is+thriving&business2=on&expanded=&x= 21&y=3.

Morgan, David. Obesity may be beginning earlier in U.S. Reuters News Service, 2002 June 17.

Murray, Bob, et al. The Uplift Program [Internet]. Depression Leads to Overeating for Women, But Not Men. [Cited in *USA Today*, 2002 March 18]: Available from: http://www.upliftprogram.com/special_h3.html#h2

Natow, Annette, et al. *Eating Out Food Counter*. New York: Pocket Books, 1998.

Netzer, Corinne T. *The Complete Book of Food Counts*. New York: Dell Publishing, 2000.

New Strategist Publications, Inc. American Men 107 Health, Chapter 4 [Internet]. [Updated 1999 May]: Available from www.newstrategist .com

Ornstein, Robert and David Sobel. *Healthy Pleasures*. Reading, MA: Addison-Wesley Publishing, 1989.

National survey reveals it takes more than sweets to satisfy young males today; From extreme sports to extreme pizza, young men indulge their intense cravings, and pizza is their food of choice. Pizza Hut press release [Internet]. 1998 October 12: Available from: http://www.pizzahut.com/pressreleases/1998/pr_news101298.asp.

Sears, Barry. *The Zone*. New York: ReganBooks, 1995.

Shapiro, Howard M. *Dr. Shapiro's Picture Perfect Weight Loss Shopper's Guide*. Emmaus, PA: Rodale Press, 2001.

Schlosser, Eric. *Fast Food Nation*. New York: Perennial/HarperCollins, 2002.

Schuler, Lou, et al. *The Testosterone Advantage Plan*. New York: Simon & Schuster/Fireside, 2003.

Smith, C. F., D. A. Williamson, et al. "Flexible vs. Rigid Dieting Strategies: Relationship with Adverse Behavioral Outcomes." *Appetite*, 32, no. 3: 295–305).

Study finds soft drink consumption up, health down. Glencoe/ McGraw-Hill [Internet]. Available from: http://www.glencoe.com/ sec/health/pdf/softdrink.pdf

Thompson, Stephanie. Food marketers introduce 'one-handed' meals; bevy of new products from portable pudding to sippy-cup soups. AdAge.com. [Internet]. 2002 May 13: Available from: http://www. adage.com/paypoints/buyArticle.cms/login?newsld=34759&auth=

Warner, Jennifer (reviewed by Smith, M.D., Michael). Super-sizing blamed for bulging waists. WebMD Medical News reviewed by Michael Smith, M.D.[Internet]. 2002 July 18: Available from:

http://my.webmd.com/content/article/48/39167.htm?lastselect-edguid={5FE84E90-BC77-4056-A91C-9531713CA348}

Warshaw, Hope S. *Guide to Healthy Restaurant Eating.* Alexandria, VA: American Diabetes Association, Inc., 2002.

Willet, Walter C. *Eat, Drink and Be Healthy: The Harvard Medical School Guide to Healthy Eating.* New York: Fireside Press, 2001.

### For Additional Information:

The American Dietetic Association [www.eatright.org]

Tufts University Health and Nutrition Newsletter [www.healthletter.tufts.edu]

Nutrition Action Newsletter Center for Science in the Public Interest [www.cspinet.org]

Centers for Disease Control and Prevention [www.cdc.gov]

The United States Department of Agriculture [www.usda.gov]

# acknowledgments

**CONNECTING THE SCIENCE** of nutrition, in all its complexity, with a marginally interested lay audience — busy and perhaps skeptical guys — necessarily required drawing on the perspectives of individuals on both sides. Fortunately I am blessed to know many people who provided knowledge, ideas, tips, rips, rants, services, pithy quotes, kitchen techniques, unflinching honesty, connections, and even confusions that inform this book. My heartfelt appreciation to each of the following:

Edward Amaral, Jr., Arlene Baguisa, Sherry Bale, Dr. Linda Bartoshuk, Kristin Beck, Philip Berger, Chad Bermingham, Eddie Besozzi, Bob Blickenstaff, Charlie Bliss, Grace Bulger, Gerry Buckley, Terry Burns, Renato Callisto, Sue Gengler Canepa, Michael Carmel, Tom Chaderjian, Danny Cohen, Jeff Conte, Thomas Conte, Marguerite Copel, Renée Zonka, Teri Denlinger, Tom Dominguez, Will Dumas, Doug Elliott, Joe Esposito (Chicago), Joe Esposito (Glen Ellyn, IL), John Faier, Keith Ferazzi, Michael Ferro, Greg Geurin, Cathy Gleason, the geniuses at Google, David Graham, Gary Gronlund, Jason Herbert, Jay Hill, Jeff Johnson, Brian Justice, Joan Horbiak, Elizabeth Karmel, Jim Kempland, Dr. Barbara Klein, Steve Knox, Kevin Kosowksi, Chris Kovich, Mark Kraniak, Tom Lawler, Bill Lederhouse, Bea Leopold, Nelson Mereles, Chris Miller, Mike Madalinski, Paul Mikos, Michael Mock, Abraham Morgentaler, Craig Nadborne, Maria Nevelson, Phil Palmer, Paul Patnode, Keith Pye, Jean Ragalie, Jason Ramos, Tom Reavis, Marty Regan, Raul Rodriguez, Lennie

Rose, Joyce Rowe, Lynn Rowley, Jeff Sachse, Eric Sanders, Dan Santow, Randy Schein, Deborah Schneider, Robert Schuckman, Mark Smithe, Dan Sproull, Jason Stidworthy, Layton Tanaka, Musa Tangoren, Nene Tovar, Kevin Voelcker, Stu Wade, Les Waite, Robert Weiner, Tom Yanney, and Todd Young.

Particular thanks go to Matthew Lore at Marlowe & Company for belief in this mission, vigorous engagement, and, together with editorial assistant Peter Jacoby, astute skill and instinct in crafting an effective message. Additionally, sincere gratitude to Deanna Conte, M.S., R.D., L.D., for her insight on both the science and psychology of guys' eating.

And finally thanks to my grandfather, the late Alex P. Klettke, who, when widowed in his 80s, learned to cook dishes like Grandma's sauerbraten; meals that sustained him another good ten years. That should prove to guys everywhere that healthy culinary skills can be acquired at any age.

—*Russ Klettke*

# index

## A

acidic juices and foods, 40, 51, 106, 117.
  *See also* vinegar
acne, processed foods and, 27
aesthetics, 143, 188–90
aging, 14, 34, 95
Agriculture, U.S. Department of, 104
airports and airplanes, 266–68
alcohol, 46–47, 82–83, 253
American Cancer Society, xxiv
American Dietetics Assn., 8, 57, 82
American Heart Assn., 96
American Medical Assn., 14, 254
antioxidants, 9, 31, 107, 113, 160
appetizers, 190–91, 222–23
Apple Peace, 211
applesauce, 211
artificial sweeteners, 48–50
artistic cooks, 139–40
Asian foods, 116, 258–59
Atkins diet, 8–9, 20, 160
attitude check, 97–98

## B

Baby Carrots, Grapes, Crackers, and
  Cheddar Cheese, 222
baking needs, purchasing, 131–33
balance, importance of, 28–29, 64, 101
bananas, 181, 239–40
barbecue grills, 128, 202, 217–20
barbecues and barbecuing
  challenges of, 215–16, 217–19
  choosing the menu, 216–17, 222–23
  non-grilled dishes, 230–40
  recipes for, 224–30
  vegetables, 219–20, 229–30
Bartoshuk, Linda, 102
Basic Beer-Can Chicken, 227–28
Basic Chicken, 177
"A Basic Review" (Karmel), 220–21
Basic Salmon, 176
Basic Skillet-Fried Steaks, 177–78
Basic Soup, 172–73
basil, 114
beans, purchasing, 133

Beck, Kirsten, 15–16
Beefnich, 209
beer, 46–47, 227–28
beverages
    calorie awareness, 46–54, 64
    for dates, 192–93
    juices, 40, 51, 106, 117
    purchasing, 132
blenders, 61, 126, 152, 153
bone density, 14
Boston Market, 59
botulism, 72
bowls, 125, 203
brand value, xxii
Brazilian Black Bean Bake, 237–38
breads, purchasing, 132–33
breakfasts, 54–56, 150–61, 244, 246–47
broccoli, 137–38, 157, 199
Broccoli Tomato Frittata, 157
Buffalo chicken wings substitute, 104
Burger King, 249
business meetings, 247, 269–70

**C**

cabbage, 239
Cajun foods, 260–61
calories
    awareness of, 9–10, 41–45, 64–65
    macronutrients and, 45–46
    McDonalds, 1950s vs. present, 16
    microneutrients and, 41
    muscle vs. fat burning of, 13–14
    restaurant vs. home dining, 8, 61,
        241–42
cancer prevention, xxiv, 9–10, 15–16, 109
canned foods, 71, 72, 133, 145–46, 167.
    *See also* tuna, canned
can opener, 123
capsaicin, 107
carbohydrates, 8–11, 24, 45–46, 92, 160.
    *See also* white carbs
cardio activity, 14
Carmel, Michael, 103
carmelizing, 105

carrots, 111, 222
car trips, 268–69
casseroles, 124, 163, 170
Center for Science in the Public
    Interest, 241–42
Centers for Disease Control, U.S., 88
cereals, 132–33, 154
Cheaters Potato Salad, 238
cheese, 86, 108, 171–72, 222, 238–39
chef's pan, 123, 163
chemicals, on or in foods, 33
chicken. *See also* smart foods
    eating out, 59–60, 63
    products made from, 12
    protein-to-fat ratio, 251
Chicken Broccoli Express, 137–38
Chicken Onion Breath, 163–64
Chicken Popeye, 167
chili, 230–31
chili peppers, 107, 113, 168–69
Chinese foods, 258–59
cholesterol, 27, 109–10
cilantro, 110
cinnamon, 111–12
citrus, Marshmallow Citrus, 240
citrus juices, 51, 106, 117
Citrus Vinaigrette, 195
cocktail buffets, 270
coconut milk, 261
coffee, 51–52, 268
colander, 126
Cold Chicken Salad, 235–36
Cole Slaw, 223
*The Color Code* (Joseph), 112–13
color of foods, 112–13, 143
complex carbohydrates, 9–10, 11
condiments, 116–17, 131–32
Conte, Deanna, 94
convenience culture. *See also* fast food
    buying into, xx, 68–71, 84–85
    healthy choices within, 82
    independence from, 93, 121–28
    predominance of, xv, 243–44
    tips to guide you through, 244–45

cooking. *See* home cooking
cooking action verbs, 147–48
cooking methods, 147–48
Cool Red Salad, 238–39
Cordain, Loren, 27
corn
    barbecuing, on the cob, 229
    as side dish, 56, 166
corn chips and salsa, 223
corn syrup, 10–11, 133
cottage cheese, 153, 180–81, 210–11
Couscous on the Loose, 201
Cracked Peppercorn Steak, 206
crackers, as appetizers, 222
cranberry relish, 115
creative food combining, 86, 115–16,
    139–40, 171–72
Creole foods, 260–61
Crunch (textures), 103–6, 114–15, 142,
    161, 191–92
cube, definition of, 148
cutting board, 125

**D**

dairy products, 12, 135
damage control, 181
Darwin's Dish, 170
dash, definition of, 147
date dinners, 187–93
deglazing, 147–48, 176
denature, 148
Denny's Restaurants, 63
depression, 94
desserts, 179–81, 193, 210–11
de-vicing, 81–86
diets
    balance within, 28–29, 64, 101
    eating smart vs., 3
    types of, xvii–xviii, 7, 34–35
Dijonnaise, 110, 116
diluting your vices, 86
*Dining Lean* (Lichten), 255–57
dinner parties, 270
dinners, 61–64, 161, 187–93, 212, 253–55

disease prevention
    cancer, xxiv, 9–10, 15–16, 109
    carbohydrates and, 9–11
    coffee and, 52
    foods for, 109–10, 113, 114, 254
    leftovers, management of, 179
    Vitamin C, 106
diseases
    acne, processed foods and, 27
    alcohol-related, 83
    diet-related, xviii, xxiii–xxiv, xxi, 41
    genetics and, 15–16
    heart disease, 96, 109–10
    kidney problems, 57
    phenylketoneuria, 49–50
    Type II Diabetes, 19
dollop, definition of, 147
Domino's Pizza, 64, 250–51
dried foods, economy of, 72

**E**

echo hunger, 24
edamame, 104–5
Edington, Dee W., 41
education and obesity, 89–90
Egg Nutrition Center, 155
eggs, 151, 252
Eggs anytime, 153
Eggs in the Pan, 156
egg substitutes, 156
*The Elements of Taste* (Kunz and
    Kaminsky), 103, 107
El Pollo Loco, 63
endocrinological effects, 24
energy drinks, 50–51
"enhanced" water, 53–54
ethnic foods, 257–65
evolution, 23–28
exercise, 7, 12, 13–16, 18, 91
experimenting with foods, 105, 146

**F**

Fancy Sweet Potatoes, 204
Faoli's Chicken Parmigiana, 63

FAQs, 33–35, 212–13
farmers' markets, 184–87
fast food. *See also* convenience culture;
    restaurants
    chicken dishes, 59–60, 63, 252
    double-fried meats, 258–59
    as dumb food, 150
    marketing of, xx
    tips for surviving, 244, 248–53
fat (body), 95–96
fat-free movement, 24
fatigue, digestion and, 9
fats (in foods)
    body's need for, 12–13, 145
    good vs. bad, 30, 92, 100–101
    metabolism and, 14, 41–42, 91, 150
    protein-to-fat ratio, 136, 151, 251–52,
        255–57
fiber, 26, 29, 43
Finland, 89–90
fish, 12, 13, 134–35, 228, 253–54. *See
    also* salmon; tuna, canned
Five Minute dishes, 153–55
flavenoids, 160
flavors. *See* tastes
flaxseed oil, 30
Food and Drug Administration (FDA),
    61, 72, 136
food industry, xix, xx–xxi, 24
food labels, reading, 136
Food Marketing Institute, 75
foods, measuring, 146–47
Four Bean Salad, 236–237
free radicals, 14
French fries, 245–46
frequency of acceptability, 85
frittatas (egg mess), 156–58
frozen foods, xvii, 32, 68–69, 71–72,
    134–35, 218–19
fruits
    berries, benefits of, 112
    for breakfast, 151–52
    caloric content of, 43–45
    in smoothies, 29, 61, 152
fruits and vegetables. *See also* fruits;
    smart foods; vegetables
    amount per day, 32–33
    benefits of, 9–10, 31, 112–13, 160
    calorie content, 51
    complex-sugar content, 25
    Cool Red Salad, 238–39
    purchasing, 131, 134
frying pans, 123, 163
functionality of tools, 130

**G**

Gaga Garbanzoaga, 171
garlic, 109–10, 168–69
Gatorade, 50–51
General Motors Corp., 41
genetics, 15–16
ginger root, 113
GirlsAtTheGrill.com, 216, 220–21,
    227–28
glop, definition of, 147
glycemic index, 11
Google.com, 146
gourmet cooking, 97–98
grains. *See* whole grains and products
green peppers, 164, 168–69, 173, 205
greens, 75, 113
green salads, 191, 193–94, 235
green tea, 52, 105
grill, George Foreman-style, 127, 175,
    202. *See also* barbecue grills
grilled vegetables, 202, 219–20
groceries, 71–72, 129–30, 131–35, 137
Guy Paradox, 88, 97–98
guys' characteristics
    cooking, 93–94
    creatures of habit, xvi
    desire to propagate species, xviii
    engineers or artists, 139–40
    food preferences, 104, 114–15
    integrity, 91–92
    intellect, 88

laissez-faire attitude, 37–38, 100
medium- and non-tasters, 102
multidimensional thinking, 92–93,
    96–97
non-obcessive, 100
team membership, 90

### H

Half Hard-Boiled Eggs, 222
Hard-Boiled Eggs, 155
health-clubs, 14–15, 61
health incentives, xviii, xxii, 5–6, 90,
    109–10, 244
heart disease, 96, 109–10
heat, stovetop cooking, 144–45
hegemonic masculinity, 90
herbs, 107, 110, 114, 198
high fructose corn syrup (HFCS),
    10–11, 133. *See also* white sugar
Hollingshead, Carolyn H., 91
home cooking
    artist vs. engineer, 139–40
    basics of, 141–48
    benefits from, 8, 61, 76–77, 105–6
    gourmet . . . not, 97–98
    kitchen preparation, 121–28
    trend toward, 75–76
    why not?, 119–20
honey, 108
Honey-Orange Bean and Vegetable
    Stew, 236
hormones, 12, 24, 83
horseradish, 110–11
Hurley, Jayne G., 241–42
hydrogenated vegetable oils, 26–27

### I

ice, in smoothies, 152
IHRSA/American Sports Data Health
    Club Trend Report 2001, 14–15
illnesses. *See* diseases
incentives. *See* health incentives
Indian foods, 261

indulgent foods, 79–86, 94
ingredients, list of on food labels, 136
Interbrand, xxi
inventory management, 137
Italian foods, 261–62

### J

Jacobson, Michael F., 241–42
Japanese foods, 259
Jeffrey, Robert, 94
jigger, definition of, 147
Joseph, James A., 112–13
juices, 40, 51, 106, 117

### K

Karmel, Elizabeth, 220–21, 227–28
Kentucky Fried Chicken, 250
kettles, 124, 172–74
kitchen preparation, 121–28
knife and knife sharpener, 124–25

### L

Labor Statistics, U.S. Bureau of, 96
Lean Cuisine, 60, 69
leftovers, 171, 175, 179, 194
lemon juice, 106
Lichten, Joanne V., 255–57
life spans, 34
Light Red Beans with Chicken,
    Oranges, and Walnuts, 207–8
lime juice, 106
lunches, 56–61, 161, 248–53
lycopene, 9, 31, 113

### M

Macaroni and Cheese with variations,
    86, 171–72
macronutrients, 26, 45–46, 100–101. *See
    also* carbohydrates; fats (in foods);
    proteins
Main Stuff, 105–6, 142–43, 161, 192
Maize Craze, 199–200
Mann, Neil, 27

marinades, 219

marketing of food products
  Dijonnaise, 110, 116
  enhanced water, 53–54
  examples of, xx, 83–85
  low-carb beer, 46

Marshmallow Citrus, 240

math, why bother with?, 37–38

mayonnaise, 116

McDonalds, 55, 58, 246, 248–49

McNamara, Donald J., 154–55

meal choices, smart vs. dumb
  breakfast, 54–56
  dinner, 61–64
  lunch, 56–61
  overview, 54

meal preparation times, 68–71

measuring foods, 146–47

meats
  beef products, 12
  cooked temperatures of, 218
  inherent dangers of, 143
  purchasing, 134–35

meat thermometers, 218

Menu Guide, protein-to-fat ratio, 255–57

menus, choosing, 216–17

menu selections, 244–45

mesclun, 193

metabolism
  capsaicin and, 107
  instinctive balancing of, 95
  thermal effect of food, 150
  weight loss and, 14, 41–42, 91

Mexican foods, 262–63

micronutrients, 26, 41

microwaves, 123, 156, 159, 225–26

Middle Eastern foods, 264–65

milk-based drinks, 53

mince, definition of, 148

Minestrone, 195–96

mixing bowl sets, 125, 203

moderation, 101, 106

monounsaturated fats, 13, 20

Mrs. Dash, 111

Multi-Bean Salad, 197–98

multidimensional thinking, 92–93, 96–97

multi-textured dishes, 103

muscles, metabolism and, 13–14

mustards, 110

**N**

National Cancer Institute, 9, 10, 109

National Institute for Consumer Research (Norway), 89–90

National Institute on Alcohol Abuse and Alcoholism, 83

*Nature* (Journal), 34

New Wave Peas 'N Eggs, 159

New York City Firefighters' weight reduction program, 89

*The New York Times*, 93

Nona Bravo's Chicken Minestrone, 195–96

North African foods, 263–64

NPR.org, 115

Nuclear Eggs, 156

Nuked Eggs, 159

Nutricize.com, 267

nutrition
  in canned and frozen foods, xiii, 71–72
  egregious acts against, 54
  food labels on, 136
  media noise, xvii
  plants and lean protein, xxii–xxiii, 31
  shopping considerations, 130
  single guys' advantage, xvi, xxiii
  variety and, 83

nuts, 131, 207–8

Nutty Bananas, 239–40

NWC (no white carbs) strategy, 10, 160–61, 168, 172

**O**

oatmeal, 55, 154

obesity epidemic

about, xviii, xxiv, 16, 27–28, 80–81
age and, 96
education, effect of, 89–90
fat-free movement and, 24
Guy Paradox, 88, 97–98
health care costs of, 41
Octopussy Pasta, 169
oils, hydrogenated vegetable, 26–27
olive oil, 20, 108–9, 145, 220
omega-3 fatty acids, 12, 30, 254
omelets vs. frittatas, 156
onions, 109, 138, 163–64
online shopping, 73–74
orange juice mixer, 126
oregano, 107
oven roasting pan, 127
Overeaters Anonymous, 80–81
overeating, 80–81, 82

**P**

Pakistani foods, 261
paper products/wraps, 135
Parmesan cheese, 108
pasta, 169, 203
Pea Garbanzo Fiesta, 200–201
peanut butter, 68–69, 95, 151, 180, 211
Peanut Butter Cabbage, 239
Peanut Butter Cottage, 210–11
Peapod.com, 73–74
peas, 68–69, 159, 166, 171
pepper, 107, 206
Pepper Fried Tuna, 164
Perricone, Nicholas, 14
*The Perricone Prescription* (Perricone),
    14
Perrier (water), 53–54
PFR (protein-to-fat ratio), 136, 151,
    251–52, 255–57
phenylketoneuria, 49–50
physical activity. *See* exercise
physiological components
    of breakfast, 150
    of color, 143
    of temptation, 270–71

phytochemicals, 9, 26, 160
pizza, 174, 233, 234–35
Plant Protein Palooza, 166
plants you can eat, 190
platitudes for friends, 117
polyunsaturated fats, 13
popcorn, temptation of, 270–71
portion control, 16–17, 82, 163
potatoes, 238, 264
potato masher, 126, 203
Powerade, 50–51
preservatives, 72
processed foods, 2, 27–28, 29. *See also*
    white carbs; white sugar
protein bars, 28, 151, 265–66
protein-based drinks, 53, 150, 265–66
Protein Egg Shakes, 151
Protein Monkey, 181
Protein Powder Shakes, 152
proteins
    awareness of, 55
    balancing quantity of, 29–30
    benefits from, xxii–xxiii, 11–13, 17
    emphasizing, 29–30
    grams per kg body weight, 57
    snacking on, 95
    toast meals with, 152
protein-to-fat ratio (PFR), 136, 151,
    251–52, 255–57
Putnam, Judith, 27

**Q**

quantity buying, 130
quasi-nutrients, 26, 160

**R**

ratios
    carbs/fats/proteins, 45–46
    protein to fat, 136, 151, 251–52,
        255–57
    vegetable to protein, 28–29, 45
raw food diets, 34–35
Red Chicken Soup, 175
restaurants. *See also* fast food

about, 8, 16, 61
breakfasts at, 244, 246–47
dinners at, 253–55
eating carbs at, 39–40
nutrition information from, 136
prices at, vs. home, 76–77
smart foods in, 241–42, 246–47
time required for dining, 69–71
tips for surviving, 244–45, 246–48
risk management, 143
roast beef dinner, PFR of, 252
Roast Chicken, 231–32
Roast Turkey, 232–33
Roberts, Ralph, 161
Roenigk, Bill, 226

**S**

saccharine, 49
salad dressings, 108, 131–32, 194–95
salads, 191, 193–94, 197–98, 235–37
salmon, 12, 251–52, 254
Salmon and Dirty Corn, 205
Salmon and Onions, 138
Salmon Cakes, 223
salsa, 114, 168, 262–63
salt, seasoning with, 107
salt substitutes, 106
sandwiches, 114–15, 161
saturated fats, 13
saucepans, 123–24, 155
Schuler, Lou, 11, 12, 91
scientific (engineers) cooks, 139–40
seafood, 169
searing, definition of, 148
Sears, Barry, 24–25
servings per container, 136
serving- vs. tablespoons, 146–47
Shapiro, Howard, 89
shelf stability, 72
shopping online, 73–74
shrimp, 62, 222
side dishes, 56, 176, 178, 191–92,
    197–204
simmer, definition of, 148

simple carbohydrates. *See* white carbs
Simple Sweet Potatoes, 204
skillets, 123, 163
slow cooking, 144
smart foods. *See also* fruits and vegeta-
    bles; health incentives; snacks and
    snacking
    about, xxii–xxiii
    acidic juices and foods, 40
    complex carbohydrates, 9–10
    evolution and, 23–28
    frozen, canned and storable, xiii,
        68–69
    healthy pizza, 233
    as only at-home option, 130
    pre-washed vegetables, xix
    in restaurants, 241–42, 246–47
    unprocessed, 19–20
smart moves. *See also* weight manage-
    ment strategies
    avoid seeing donut shops, 85
    de-vicing, 81–86
    distract yourself with low-cal food,
        17, 86
    filling up with produce, xxii–xxiii,
        30, 32–33, 39
    home cooking, 8
    savor small quantities, 19
    shift gradually to substitutes, 19
    smaller plate, 17
    substitute vegetables for simple
        carbs, 39–40
    weight management, 5–6, 8–21,
        28–29, 45, 88–97
smoothies, 29, 61, 152
snacks and snacking
    benefits of, 17–18, 94
    instincts about, 94, 95
    suggestions for, 18, 40, 160–61, 245,
        268–69
    superiority of protein, 95
sodas, 47, 48–50, 97
soups, 133–34, 172, 191, 230–31
spices, 107, 111–12, 206

spicy garden mix, 113
spinach, 75, 167, 209
spoons, table vs. serving, 146–47
spoons and spatulas, 125–26
sports, 4, 90
sports drinks, 50–51
Stamberg, Susan, 115
Starbucks, 52
Steak, barbecuing, 225
steak sauces, 111
steamer insert, 124, 197–98
stews, 236
stir-fry, definition of, 147
stockpots. *See* kettles
stomach space, 38–40, 64
stovetop cooking, 144–45
structure, importance of
    balance, variety and moderation, 101
    impressing women with, 187
    occasional indulgences, 94
    quality of, xvi
    taking control of, 75–76
    whole-life approach, 96–97
Subway, 58, 252–53
sugar. *See* high fructose corn syrup;
    white sugar
sun-dried tomatoes, 113, 167, 199–200
*Supermarket News*, 84
Sushi, 259
sweeteners, 108. *See also* white sugar
Sweet Potato Chicken Soup, 196–97
sweet potatoes, 203, 204

**T**

Tabasco, 107
Taco Bell, 249–50
Taco Fresco, 59
taste preferences, 103
tastes (flavors)
    Four Bean Salad, 236–37
    guys' favorites, 106–14
    pain/pleasure relative to, 102
    as part of complete meal, 142–43
    personal nature of, 101–2

for sandwiches, 161
sense of smell and, 115
in side dishes, 191–92
smart food tastes good, 99–101
taste transfers, 104–5, 111
tea, 51–52, 105
team membership, 90
TEF (thermal effect of food), 150
temptation, physiological component
    of, 270–71
tenderize, definition of, 148
testosterone, 12, 83
*The Testosterone Advantage Plan*
    (Schuler), 11, 12, 91
Teutonic Corn, 200
textures. *See* Crunch
Thai foods, 259–60
thermal effect of food, 150
time required for meal preparation,
    68–71, 149–50
toaster, 128
toast meals, 152
tomatoes, 9, 31, 104, 113
Tomato Fiesta Soup, 173
Tomato Potato, 203
total fat and types (food labels), 136
transfatty acids, 27, 92–93, 100
travel, challenges of, 266–70
tuna, canned, 56, 162, 164–66, 168, 254
Tuna Louisiana, 168
Tuna-on-the-Hoof, 165–66
turbo-cooker, 127–28
Turkey, Roast, 232–33
Turkey Burgers, 224
Turkey Chili, 230–31

**V**

Vampire Be Gone Chicken, 168–69
variety, balance and moderation, 101
vegetables. *See also* fruits and vegetables
    convenient, xv, 113
    cooking, 145, 176, 219–20, 229–30
    filling up with, xxii–xxiii, 30, 32–33, 39
    vegetable to protein ratio, 28–29, 45

vices, chronic, 79–81
Vietnamese foods, 260
vinegar, 40, 106–7, 113, 194–95
Viva Bean Frittata, 158

**W**

walnuts, crushing, 208
water, 50–51, 53–54
watermelon, 43
weight, 4, 7, 15–16. *See also* obesity epi-
    demic
weight lifting, 14
weight management, 5–6, 8–21, 28–29,
    45, 88–97. *See also* smart moves
Wendy's (fast food), 249
whey-protein concentrates, 12, 53
white carbs
    about, 10–11, 25, 40
    in ethnic foods, 260, 262, 264
    NWC strategy, 10, 46, 160–61, 168,
        172
    obesity epidemic and, 27–28
white sugar, 10–11, 48–50, 52–53, 53–54.
    *See also* high fructose corn syrup
whole grains and products
    benefits from, 10, 34, 160
    human evolution and, 23–24
    pasta, 169, 203

percent of on plate, 46
    purchasing, 132–33
Wild Rice and Broccoli, 199
Wild West Pizza, 234–35
wines, 192–93
women
    FAQs about, 212–13
    farmers' markets and, 184–87
    guys' differences from, 88, 91–92
    recipes for success with, 193–213
    super- and medium-tasters, 102
    why cook for?, 94, 183–84
workouts, pre- and post-, 17–18, 67–68,
    265–66

**Y**

Yin Yang Yogurt/Applesauce, 211
yogurt, 111, 151, 153, 180, 181, 211
Yogurt and Fruit, 153
Yogurt/Applesauce Mix, 180
Yogurt/Peanut Butter Pull, 180, 211
yo-yo effect, 14

**Z**

Zone diet, 7, 8, 24–25, 28–35, 160
*The Zone* (Sears), 24–25
Zonka, Renée, 115